THE

W9-DJQ-904

NURSING HOME PRIMER

A Comprehensive Guide to Nursing Homes
and Other Long-Term Care Options

Hanns G. Pieper, Ph.D.

BETTERWAY PUBLICATIONS, INC.
WHITE HALL, VIRGINIA

Published by Betterway Publications, Inc.
Box 219
Crozet, VA 22932

Cover design by Tim Haley
Typography by Typecasting
Photographs:
(1) taken by Susan Riley at The Cedars Nursing Home, Char-
lottesville, Virginia; (2) courtesy of Margaret Thacker, The
Cedars Nursing Home; (3) courtesy of Dr. Hanns G. Pieper.

This book has been written to provide useful information to
persons considering selection of a nursing home or other long
term care facility for a family member or friend. Readers are
encouraged to seek professional advice during the decision-
making process.

Library of Congress Cataloging-in-Publication Data

Pieper, Hanns Gunter,
    The nursing home primer: a consumer's guide for the
elderly and their families / Hanns G. Pieper.

        p.   cm.
    Includes index.
    ISBN 1-55870-115-X: $7.95
    1. Nursing homes. 2. Consumer education. I. Title.
RA997.P54   1989
362.1'6'0880565 — dc19   88–37712
                                                 CIP

Printed in the United States of America
0 9 8 7 6 5 4 3 2 1

*I would like to dedicate this book to my wife, my son,
my daughter and my parents, all of whom
have brought great joy to my life.*

ACKNOWLEDGMENTS

This book is a summary of materials and lectures that I have presented in my classes, in workshops for careproviders, public seminars, and counseling sessions. Some of the insights come from my own research and practice but I also am indebted to the work of my fellow gerontologists who have conducted research which has helped us in our understanding of the nature of institutionalization and nursing home care.

I am also indebted to the many nursing home staff members who have taken time to talk with me about nursing home care over the past ten years.

Finally, I would like to acknowledge a debt to ten very special nursing home residents who took a great deal of time to meet with me over a period of four months during my sabbatical to gather practical insights in preparation for this book. These persons — Louise, Aurelia, Norma, Cleo, Betty, Bertha, Helen, Edna, Bill and Al — took the time to offer their insights and the benefit of their experience to help ease the introduction to nursing home life for future residents and their families. It is my great hope that this book succeeds in that aim.

CONTENTS

CHAPTER 1

Evaluating the Situation

If you are reading this book you are probably faced with the difficult question of whether or not a family member or friend should be placed in a nursing home. No one needs to tell you how emotionally draining this situation is and how much you want to make the right decision.

You are not alone. Hundreds of thousands of other people will also be faced with this problem this year, but the decision remains a lonely and difficult one. Most people have no experience in choosing a nursing home, and have very little information to guide them. As you know, nobody can make the decision for you.

The purpose of this book is to provide basic information about selecting a nursing home, moving into the home and adjusting to nursing home life. The information provided should be combined with information from other sources such as health care professionals, clergy, social workers or geriatric counselors as you proceed with your deliberations.

Each chapter provides information about a specific topic and stands on its own, but you are encouraged to read the entire book to derive the maximum benefit from the materials which have been presented. In addition to this brief general introduction to the book, this chapter explores some of the questions which must be answered when making the decision to move into a nursing home.

The vast majority of nursing home residents are women, and usually their adult children (mostly daughters) help them find a good nursing home. To simplify the writing style and avoid the cumbersome "he/she" I have assumed that you are looking for a nursing home for your mother and have adjusted the style accordingly. Of course, almost everything that applies to a mother also applies to a father.

I have also assumed that your mother is not bedfast and that, while she may be somewhat disoriented, she has retained some of her abilities to function mentally. This assumption was made because this kind of person would require the widest range of social and psychological services; therefore most social and psychological needs will be covered. Important exceptions to this general assumption are discussed in several places in the book.

A BIG DECISION

Now let us turn our attention to the question of whether or not an elderly person should move into a nursing home. Actually, this question really contains a number of questions. The first question and the one that is addressed in the rest of this chapter is whether or not the elderly person can continue to live independently. If the answer to this question is "no," the older person must ask herself if one of the alternatives discussed in chapter two will meet her needs or whether a nursing home is necessary. If the latter is the case, the decision must be made as to which nursing home will be best.

The question of whether or not an elderly person can continue to live independently in her own home may develop over a long period of time as it becomes more and more obvious that managing alone at home is becoming increasingly difficult. On the other hand, the question may come with bewildering swiftness following an illness or injury.

When the time comes to reach a decision concerning the question of continued independent living, *whose* decision are we talking about? The answer depends in a large part on your mother's mental ability and her willingness to assume responsibility for the decision. If your mother is no longer able to function clearly mentally, then much of the burden of the decision will fall upon you, but if your mother still functions well mentally, it is her decision as much as anybody's. Sometimes we middle-aged children tend to forget this in our zeal to provide what we think is the safest and best possible environment for our parents.

Gerontologists agree that the potential nursing home resident should be involved in as many phases of the decision making as possible. After all, it is a major decision that will affect how that person will spend the rest of her life. In all likelihood it will be emotionally difficult to discuss moving into a nursing home with your mother, but many problems can be avoided through her involvement at this most important juncture in her life.

We all like to feel that we have some control over our lives, and this is particularly important for older persons who often feel that much control has slipped away from them. Being involved makes it your mother's decision as well as yours, and she has retained some control over her destiny. This appears to have an impact on adjustment to the home: it has been shown that nursing home residents who have been actively involved in the decisions leading to the move generally adjust to their new environment much more quickly and more positively than those who had not been involved.

Going about making the decision in a systematic way will help you to reach the most appropriate conclusion, and will probably help you and your mother feel more positive about the decision once it has been made.

YOUR MOTHER'S HEALTH

As in any situation where a decision has to be made, the best way to begin is by gathering as much information as possible. Probably the most important thing to determine is the degree to which your mother is no longer able to function. A thorough physical examination is the first step. It is quite possible that the problem which has you considering the possibility of a nursing home is due to a physical ailment which can be cleared up. For instance, nutritional deficiencies are thought to be related to a host of problems, including some forms of memory loss.

Be sure that the examining physician is aware of all the medications your mother is taking. Drug interactions may cause confusion, depression, or a multitude of other problems which can be straightened out by prescribing more compatible medicines. Do not assume that your physician is aware of all of your mother's medications unless she is only treated by that particular physician and no other. Any over-the-counter drugs your mother is using should also be considered at this time. One way of dealing with potential drug interactions is to buy all prescription drugs from the same pharmacy, so that pharmacists can spot conflicting drug prescriptions. The examination should also include an assessment of hearing and vision, since treatable sensory losses can often lead to behavioral problems.

If possible, the examination should be performed by a physician with a specialty in geriatric medicine, one who is aware of the unique health problems of older persons. Otherwise treatable diseases such as depression can be and often are dismissed as part of the normal aging process by physicians who are not sensitive.

You should also make an inventory of your mother's physical and mental skills. Make a list of activities that are a necessary part of her normal daily routines, and rate them according to the degree to which she can perform each one. Begin by looking at the two biggest danger areas in most homes, the kitchen and the bathroom. For instance, can she cook, get food off the shelves, wash dishes? Has she ever left food cooking on the range and forgotten about it? Can she use the toilet, get into the bathtub, and clean the bathroom? How about other daily activities, such as washing clothes or making beds? Does she have difficulty moving from room to room? Does she have easy access to phones? Does she have confused periods when she wanders aimlessly in the neighborhood? Does she take her medication regularly? Can she manage her own financial affairs? What kinds of medical care does she require?

Include as many things on the list as you possibly can. Then order the items according to (1) those that are absolutely necessary for safety and survival, (2) those which are important to maintain an adequate lifestyle and finally (3) those which help make life more pleasant but which are not absolutely necessary. Share your information and conclusions with someone — your family physician, a social worker from the local Council on Aging, or the director of the local hospital or a local nursing home. Together you should be able to reach the most appropriate decision.

In general, not being able to perform the activities in the first category would, of course, be reason for concern and for considering one of the alternatives discussed in the next chapter. If, after matching your mother's level of impairment with the services provided by the alternatives, it appears that they will meet her needs without institutionalization, those alternatives should be vigorously explored. If the alternatives are unavailable or impractical or if they simply do not meet your mother's needs, then the nursing home may be the most appropriate choice. If your mother really needs a nursing home, none of the alternatives mentioned will meet her needs as well. Gerontological studies have shown that when senior citizens really need the services of a nursing home, moving into such a home can have a very positive impact on both life satisfaction and physical health.

CHAPTER 2

Noninstitutional Services

Sometimes even when an elderly person can no longer live in her present home, a nursing home is not necessarily the next most practical choice. In this chapter we will look at some other services that may meet your mother's needs. These services are often called alternatives to nursing home care, but use of the term *alternatives* may be a bit misleading. If a person really needs the services of a nursing home, there are no alternatives.

However, the services discussed in this chapter could be used by many persons who presently reside in nursing homes. It is certainly appropriate to determine if any of these services will meet your requirements before you proceed with the move into the nursing home. Gerontologists estimate that at least one-fourth of all present nursing home residents would not need to be in the nursing home if these other services were available and utilized. Chart 2–1 presents the alternatives and services in order from least supportive to most supportive. Each of these alternatives is briefly discussed in this chapter. The discussion of each service is preceded by a short vignette to illustrate the type of problem the service addresses. While the illustrations are purely imaginary, they are quite typical and realistic.

Before we look at these service alternatives, we should look at one subject which almost always comes up during family nursing home discussions, the subject of having Mom move in with one of the children. In the past it was a relatively common practice for Mom to move in with an unmarried daughter who assumed the responsibility for her care.

MOTHER MOVING IN

Having Mother move in with you may be a great solution or an absolutely terrible one. It is an arrangement best approached with much thought and caution, because it usually involves a radical change in lifestyle for your mother as well as you and your family.

Alternatives	Support Systems
Living in original home	Emergency Call Systems
	Adult Day Care
E.C.H.O. Housing	Respite Care
	Senior Centers
Shared Housing	Meals on Wheels
	Public Meal Program
Boarding Homes	Home Health Care
	Friendly Visitor
Retirement Centers	Telephone Reassurance
	Homemaker Services
Congregate Housing	Equity Conversions
	Home Renovations
Residential Housing	Live-In
Living with Family	
Intermediate Nursing Home	
Skilled Nursing Home	

Chart 2-1   Housing Alternatives

There are many practical things which have to be considered. For starters, take a good look at your home. Is it large enough to accommodate an additional adult? Not only will an extra bedroom be needed, but the bathroom, kitchen, and family rooms will also be more used.

Aside from the space considerations there are the social factors. How will a three-generation family living together affect social relationships in the family? Inevitably there will be a loss of privacy, because your mother cannot be expected to remain in isolation all day. This loss of privacy will affect everyone in the household. You will probably feel much more constrained in some interactions with your children or spouse. Your mother will also feel the loss of privacy; many older persons prefer to retain as much independence as possible by living as independently as they can.

To what extent are the lifestyles of all the generations compatible? By the time we are adults we are all pretty well settled into certain ways of doing things, and there are thousands of things we can do to get on each other's nerves. It is just not realistic to expect anyone to really change his or her lifestyle. You might ask yourself how things went the last time you were together for a long period of time. To put it rather bluntly, if you couldn't wait to get back home or were counting the hours until she went back home, there may be potential problems.

If the parent requires medical or custodial care, some concerns must be faced. Do family caregivers have the abilities or the time to provide the necessary care? If the problem becomes worse will the family be able to handle the new responsibilities?

This is a time for a frank and honest discussion involving everyone who will be living in the household. You should feel comfortable in saying that you don't think it will work out without feeling guilty, and your mother should feel comfortable in saying that she doesn't think it will work out without feeling that you think she is ungrateful for your efforts.

This discussion may sound somewhat pessimistic. In many situations multigenerational households work out beautifully. However, living together under the wrong circumstances can result in years of conflict and tension, and may have a negative impact on your relationship with your mother and your family. If you don't feel you can live together, remember that there are many other excellent service alternatives available.

If, after examining all sides of the question, both you and your mother agree that you can live together, that's great. If it is obvious that this is not the best solution, it is better to discover this before your presently good relationship deteriorates due to the stresses of living together. You still have a good relationship with your mother, and you can build upon it by finding other suitable means of meeting your mother's needs.

You may find that friends and even other family members (who often didn't want Mom moving in with them either) will react negatively to your decision not to have Mother move in with you. At these times it often helps to remember that it was you and your mother's decision and that no matter how well-meaning your friends may be, they do not have your knowledge of all of the factors involved and they will not have to live with any of the consequences of the decision. There are many other alternatives which may be able to provide your mother with the care she requires. Let's now turn our attention to these alternatives.

CASE #1

Hazel has lived in her home for over fifty years. Her general health is pretty good but she is experiencing some of the sensory losses which happen to all of us as we grow older. Her daughter Lola is worried that these losses may result in a serious accident and has suggested that Hazel move to a nursing home or a senior citizen's apartment near Lola's house. Hazel is absolutely adamant that she will not move from her home.

Lola's problem is quite common. Even though her mother refuses to move, Lola still has some options. One of the most important of these is to do what she can to prevent an accident by making her mother's home safer. Actually making the home safer is a pretty good idea under any circumstances. Accidents are an ever present threat for older persons and often result in injuries which make institutionalization necessary. The changes should be made *before* an accident occurs.

Just exactly what Lola should do depends upon what sensory problems her mother is experiencing, but there are some general recommendations. Many of the things she can do are inexpensive, such as increasing the wattage of the light bulbs in the house. Many older persons require much more light to see the same things that a younger person can see. Experiments have demonstrated that differences in visual ability between younger and older persons can be reduced when older persons are provided with more light. Caution should be exercised to be sure that the wattage capacity of the fixture is not exceeded.

Because older persons often don't lift their feet as high as younger persons when they walk, scatter rugs should be removed and floor surfaces should be as flat as possible. Irregularities in floor surfaces which cannot be removed should be clearly marked so they can be seen easily. Louder door bells and telephone ringers can be installed to make sure they are heard. Devices for telephones which help the person hear better are also available and easy to install. The installation of additional phones throughout the house may also make life easier and certainly make it easier to summon help in an emergency.

In multifloor houses it may be helpful to rearrange the home so that all activity can take place on one level. This may require some major renovations if bathrooms and washing machines have to be relocated. It may mean that a room formerly used for some other purpose may become a bathroom / clothes washing area.

Often major renovations are needed in the kitchen and bathroom areas. These two rooms are particularly dangerous areas and the locations of many serious accidents. Bars fastened to room walls and in the shower can help prevent a dangerous fall. If losing balance is a frequently occurring problem, bars should also be installed in hallways. Kitchens can be rearranged to minimize stretching or the necessity of having to climb on things to reach higher shelves. Some people suggest installing a microwave oven in the place of more dangerous gas stoves. Microwave ovens also turn themselves off, an important feature when forgetfulness is a problem.

Sometimes it helps to replace some of the furniture with more supportive furniture. As the years progress, it may become more difficult to get out of the old overstuffed couch or chair. These can be replaced by a firmer yet just as comfortable chair. Chairs which gently raise the occupant to a standing position can be purchased at stores which sell or rent convalescent aids.

Some of these changes are easily and cheaply accomplished. Others may require extensive and perhaps rather expensive remodeling. However, the cost of such renovations may be less than the cost of spending just a month in a nursing home. Most importantly, the renovations may help avoid the injuries which can ruin the later years of life.

ALTERNATIVE HOUSING

CASE #2

Ellie is in marginal health and has been living by herself since her husband Frank died four years ago. She has a nice home, but it is large and she no longer has the physical strength to do the necessary cleaning and upkeep. Heating and cooling costs are also a major problem. For these and a number of other reasons it is clear that she really cannot stay in her home but should move to a more supportive environment. Ellie recognizes her difficulties.

Ellie is one of those difficult borderline cases. She can't continue to live safely by herself, but she really does not require the services of a nursing home. What she needs is a supportive environment in which she can make the best use of her abilities. A number of alternatives may help in such a situation. The first of these is often referred to as *congregate housing*.

Congregate housing is designed specifically for older persons. It usually takes the form of efficiency apartments which contain a kitchen, bathroom, and a large living/bedroom. Some are also available in one to two bedroom apartments. The apartments are specially constructed to compensate for some of the losses in functioning which accompany aging. For instance, the kitchens have safe appliances and are designed so that shelves are within easy reach. Features include bathrooms with railings and other safety measures such as call buttons. Entry to the building may be limited and supervised so that only residents and their guests may have access. The owners of congregate housing must supply one communal activity each day. Usually that is the noon meal. Some congregate apartment complexes also provide regularly scheduled leisure activities. Often housekeeping services are also available. With the important exceptions of the increased safety and comfort, living in congregate housing does not differ a great deal from life in any other apartment.

Congregate housing is available in all price ranges. For individuals with modest financial resources, low income subsidized housing for older persons exists in many communities. Various organizations such as churches and civic groups sponsor congregate housing, and many have sliding rent scales which adjust to the financial resources of the tenant. Many cities also have more expensive luxury apartments with the same safety and convenience features.

Usually the rent for congregate housing is paid on a monthly basis with no required payments before moving in. However, the financial commitments should be thoroughly explored before moving.

If you are seriously considering a particular congregate housing arrangement, be sure to ask the manager what their policy is concerning moving out of the housing unit. One of the problems facing many congregate housing units at this time is that residents who entered in reasonably good physical and mental health have become progressively more debilitated over the years. These persons are no longer really suited to congregate housing and require even more support. Policies on moving out vary greatly. For instance, some units ask residents to move out if they become wheelchair-bound while others allow residents to stay as long as they can adequately care for themselves, even if they require nurses to live with them.

A particularly desirable form of housing is *phased housing*. Phased housing is a special arrangement which includes congregate type residential housing as well as intermediate and skilled nursing home facilities in the same general location. The two types of housing are totally separate, but they are physically close enough for easy access from one to the other. The real advantage of such an arrangement can be seen in a situation where a couple has lived in congregate housing, but one partner later develops an illness which requires a move into a nursing home. In other circumstances this could cause a lot of disruption and it might be very difficult for the couple to see each other, but living in phased housing can ease what might otherwise be a disastrous situation. In a typical phased housing complex, the entry to the complex is controlled for the safety of residents by having a gatekeeper at the only entrance. The residential housing is situated around the perimeter with most of the individual housing units containing four apartments. A few larger housing units are also provided. The intermediate and skilled care units are centrally located. Occupants of the private housing units have access to the resources of both the skilled and intermediate care units. The entire complex is fenced in at a discreet distance to provide for the security of residents. For rural areas where land is readily available, this arrangement would be ideal, but it would be somewhat impractical in urban areas. However, a similar effect could be achieved by building up rather than out and designating certain wings or floors as private residential housing, intermediate, and skilled housing.

Board and care homes are also making a comeback of sorts. These homes are extensions of the boarding homes which were found in many localities years ago. However, board and care homes are licensed. They provide the basics — a room, housekeeping, meals and, depending on the home, some degree of protective supervision. Many board and care homes are private residences owned by individuals or couples, but larger board and care homes owned and managed by corporations also exist. Charges in these homes are generally not compensated by public or private insurance.

People who want an environment with more services and who have more money to spend may find what they are looking for in *retirement villages.* Retirement villages can take the form of whole towns where occupancy is limited to retired persons, or of more familiar retirement housing complexes in cities. These complexes frequently include shops, recreational facilities such as golf courses, restaurants, and a host of other services.

Because retirement villages rarely have to conform to established standards, financial agreements vary greatly from one retirement center to another. Sometimes the resident simply buys the apartment and is then entitled to all of the other services. The apartment may become a part of the resident's estate or it may revert back to the retirement center upon the resident's death or if the resident should decide to leave. Some centers require a substantial payment in the beginning and then charge a flat rental rate for the duration of the stay. Sometimes certain rental rates are guaranteed for the entire length of the stay. The variations seem to be endless and should be thoroughly understood before any contracts or leases are signed. Again, it is important to determine when your mother would have to move out, should her health grow worse.

CASE #3

Emily was widowed about a year ago. She and her husband Bill never owned a home but they built up a tidy savings account and she is financially secure. Emily has been very lonely since Bill's death and she would enjoy living with other older persons but she is not at all interested in any kind of formal institutional arrangement.

Emily has an interesting, newly-developing option called *shared housing.* In this housing arrangement several older persons live in the same house and share certain parts of it such as the living room, dining room and kitchen, but also have a private room of their own. Some shared housing is owned and supported by civic groups in the community or run by local governments. It is also possible for the tenants to jointly own the house in which they live. The advantages of shared housing include shared costs and companionship. This is probably the least developed of all the housing alternatives, but it surely has the greatest promise as a cost-effective housing alternative for older persons.

CASE #4

Janet's mother can no longer live alone at her home. Neither Janet nor her mother find a nursing home-type environment attractive and because they live in a rural area, they don't have ready access to congregate or other supportive housing. The nearest suitable housing arrangement is over 70 miles away. Janet's mother has suggested the possibility of her moving in with Janet. While Janet and her mother get along wonderfully experience has taught Janet that when they are together in the same house for an extended period of time, friction begins to develop between them. As a result she is really hesitant about her mother moving in, but there really does not seem to be an alternative.

This is a difficult situation but perhaps one answer to Janet's problem might be E.C.H.O. (Elder Cottage Housing Opportunity) housing. This is temporary housing which is placed near the home of a caregiver such as a child or other family member. E.C.H.O. housing is completely self-contained, does not physically become a part of the main residence on the property, and thus has its own entrance. Most housing of this type is pre-manufactured and is reusable since it can be moved easily from lot to lot.

It provides privacy for both parties yet assistance is always nearby, and there is ample opportunity to get together and chat. E.C.H.O. housing is particularly suitable for rural areas where house lots are often larger and zoning restrictions are not quite so constraining.

Life care or *continuing care* arrangements were very popular a number of years ago and again seem to be enjoying growth. Life care arrangements differ considerably, but basically they involve turning over one's assets in return for a guarantee of having all of one's needs taken care of for the rest of one's life. This includes housing, social, psychological, and medical needs. Life care arrangements should be approached with extreme caution because they involve a considerable risk. In the past, life care providers have underestimated the cost of care for residents, gone broke, and left the residents without any means of support. It is important to realize that in most life care communities the residents really do not own anything, including the apartment in which they live.

This doesn't mean the idea is all bad, just that the consumer should be very careful and ask a lot of questions. It is important to determine how solid the financial base is and how much reserve the life care community has accumulated. Find out what services are covered by the fee and what extra services will have to be paid for. Is the nursing home component of the life care community Medicare and Medicaid approved? Determine what kinds of medical care will be covered by your contract and also if there is a limit to the amount of care that the life care community will provide.

Since most life care arrangements involve a hefty up-front payment, in addition to monthly fees, determine how much of the up-front payment is refundable should you decide to move out. Another important financial consideration relates to the fees. Determine if the monthly fees can go up in future years, and if so, is there a cap or limit as to how much they can increase? Because there are so many factors involved, it is essential that competent professional help be sought before signing on the dotted line.

SUPPORT SYSTEMS

CASE #5

Bob's widowed father has been living by himself and managing reasonably well. However, he has recently developed an illness which requires regular but not around-the-clock medical care. Over the past month it has become obvious to Bob that his father is neglecting the medical procedures ordered by the doctor. He is afraid that a nursing home where his father's care will be supervised is the only solution to the problem.

CASE #6

Emma's mother recently had an operation. The operation went well, but Emma has been told that her mother faces a long period of recuperation during which she will need help with most of her daily needs. Emma lives 650 miles away and a nursing home is being considered.

CASE #7

This past April, Joan's mother-in-law celebrated her eightieth birthday. The children, all of whom live out of town, planned a big family reunion at Grandma's. Joan volunteered to visit Grandma early and prepare everything for the reunion. Although Joan and her family had visited over Christmas, she was not prepared for what she found when she arrived. While Grandma had been an impeccable housekeeper, the house could only be described as dirty. Joan found that even though her mother-in-law was still mentally sharp, her physical stamina had declined considerably. She was simply not able to continue doing the work necessary to keep her large house clean.

In Bob's case complex medical care is required. In Emma's there is a need for ongoing rehabilitative assistance and in Joan's the needs are basically housekeeping needs. The situations just described vary considerably, but in all cases the families might be able to benefit from *home health care providers*. Home health care providers have been around for almost a century, but because of recent attempts to control the dramatic increase in health care costs, home health care providers have enjoyed significant growth. Home health care services can be divided into two broad areas — nursing care and homemaker services.

Nursing services include care required for chronic ilnesses such as diabetes or arthritis, as well as such services as ostomy care, catheters, medications, and injections. Therapy is available for rehabilitation from strokes, fractures, and many kinds of surgery where full recovery requires physical therapy. The expertise of occupational therapists is available to help people return to a normal lifestyle. Social workers are available to help individuals obtain community support services in addition to providing direct sevices such as counseling.

Homemaker services include shopping, meal planning, meal preparation, child care, and housekeeping. These services are provided on a regular basis by individuals who come into the home several times a day. Some agencies also offer what is frequently called *companion sitter services*. In this situation a

trained live-in person does light housekeeping, shopping, pre-
pares meals, and sees that medication is taken at the appropriate
time.

Home health care is available from a number of sources. In
some states it is provided by public health departments. Not-for-
profit agencies as well as private for-profit agencies provide care
in most localities. These providers differ considerably in structure, but as a consumer you will probably not notice much difference in either the nature or the quality of the services actually provided.

Few home health care agencies will provide all of the services
discussed above, and prices will vary from agency to agency.
Therefore, some shopping around is usually necessary to find the
agency that provides the needed care at the best price. Some
things to consider include making sure that the agency is licensed
by the state, is Medicare certified, and provides all the services
you need at the present time or are likely to need in the future.
The latter is important with some diseases like diabetes which
may require higher levels of care as the disease progresses. Moving
around from agency to agency can be disrupting to the patient.

The agency should provide you with a written total health
care plan which lists all of the services to be provided for you,
describes the purpose of each service, and lists the total cost of
each service. Agencies will not be able to provide you with this
information until they are aware of all the services which they
will be providing. This cannot usually be done until they have
checked with your doctor, so don't expect to get an estimate over
the phone. Sometimes an insurer will pay for only a certain
amount of care or for a certain amount of time. You should
check with your insurance agent to find out if this is true in your
case, and determine how the payment will be covered when the
insurer stops paying.

Home health care can be paid for in many ways. Most private group insurance companies, health maintenance organizations, and public programs such as Medicare will now pay for
many home health care services, particularly those which are
medically related. Some of the expenses may be out-of-pocket,
but many agencies have sliding fee scales which automatically
adjust the cost of the service to the consumer's income and ability
to pay.

Determining how to pay for home health care services can be
a most confusing matter for anyone. Often this involves putting

together a package consisting of government and private insurance programs. Hospital or health care agency social workers
should be reliable guides in leading you through this maze.

CASE #8

Janice's mother has recently been released from the hospital
and is receiving follow-up care from a home health care agency.
While Janice is satisfied that her mother is receiving the necessary medical care, she is concerned about her mother's welfare
because she knows that her mother is still not able to do many
things for herself. For instance, in an emergency her mother
might not be able to call for help. Unfortunately, the home
health care agency does not provide a companion service and
Janice works and lives in another state. She has been calling
her mother several times a day, but on her income Janice cannot keep this up for long.

There are several programs which might be helpful in situations where the basic need is for regular monitoring of an older
person's welfare. *Telephone reassurance programs* provide for a
daily (or more frequent if necessary) phone call to the elderly
person. Usually the agency providing this service will call the
person at an agreed-upon time of the day. If the person does not
answer or needs assistance, a designated relative or friend will be
notified by the agency and that person can then decide what to do.

Many areas also offer *emergency call systems.* In many ways
this is even better than the telephone reassurance service. With
this service the individual carries a small transmitter which is
usually attached to the belt or pinned to a blouse, and if help is
needed she simply pushes a button. A message will be received
by the agency sponsoring the program. The agency will then
either provide help or summon those who will. This service is
ideal because it provides an immediate response. It also deals
directly with one of the major fears of many older persons living
alone, which is sustaining a serious injury such as a hip fracture
and not being able to get to a phone. Another advantage is that
it does not commit people to be near a phone at a certain time of
the day. Its drawback is that it does not provide the person-to-
person interaction that many older persons enjoy.

Person-to-person interaction can be provided through another program called the *friendly visitor* program. This program, which is frequently sponsored by churches and staffed by volunteers, provides for regularly scheduled visits. While friendly visitors provide very important social stimulation, they generally do not provide any other services.

CASE #9

Henry's mother lives alone and is really managing quite well. He visits his mother quite frequently because they live in the same town. On his last visit he tried to fix himself a lunch and found mostly "junk food" in the pantry. While discussing the lack of nutritious food with his mother he discovered that her diet was seriously lacking in a balance of healthy foods.

Henry's mother is typical of many elderly persons who don't get the necessary vitamins and minerals to maintain good health. There are many reasons why older persons cease to eat nutritious meals. Sometimes the taste buds have degenerated to the point where "normal" foods just don't have any taste. Many persons who live alone don't bother to fix meals because it's simply no fun to eat alone. Maintaining a good diet is absolutely essential since it affects not only physical health but also mental health. Some forms of memory loss, for instance, are thought to be related to dietary deficiencies.

One solution to this problem may be the *Meals on Wheels* program. This private service provides a nutritious hot meal once a day, usually five days a week. Since the meals are delivered in person by a volunteer, the program also indirectly provides some social interaction. There is also a safety feature associated with *Meals on Wheels* because of the daily contact. Usually the volunteers who deliver the food are instructed to notify their office if a person does not answer the door and has not notified the agency about not being at home. Costs for the meals are very low but are paid for by the consumer.

Many areas also have publicly funded *nutrition programs.* Meals are usually distributed through these programs at senior citizen centers or restaurants which contract to provide the meals. Often there is no charge for qualifying senior citizens, although donations are usually accepted.

CASE #10

Helen moved in with her daughter Jenny and her family two years ago. Things have worked out pretty well and Helen gets along well with her son-in-law. The only real problem is that Jenny and her husband hate to leave Helen alone and have not had a social evening to themselves since Helen moved in.

Getting a break from the routine is essential to maintaining a good outlook toward life and is especially important in situations such as Jenny's. A *respite program* may provide the answer to Jenny's dilemma. Respite programs provide temporary care. The length of the service may range from a few hours to as much as several weeks while the family caregivers go on an extended vacation. In some cases someone comes to stay with the elderly person. Some nursing homes provide respite care for periods of time ranging from an afternoon to several weeks. During this time the services provided by the nursing home are available to the respite care consumer. Paying for respite care is usually an out-of-pocket expense.

CASE #11

Three years ago Henry's mother Bertha moved in with his family. At the time things worked out very well. However, Henry's wife is planning to resume her career. This means that nobody will be home to stay with Bertha and neither Henry nor his wife feel that Bertha can stay home by herself. They are considering a nursing home, but would prefer another solution.

The *adult day care center* may be the solution to Henry's problem. As the name implies, these centers provide care for older persons during the working day. The family care-giver takes the older person to the center on the way to work and picks her up on the way home in the evening.

Adult day care centers provide services ranging from the purely recreational to the therapeutic. For instance, centers may provide general nursing services, social work services, meals, nutritional counseling, recreational services, speech therapy, physical therapy, rehabilitative services, music therapy, reality therapy, and transportation services.

Day care centers are not the same as senior citizen centers. Senior citizen centers are places where older persons can get together and perhaps participate in some planned programs. Day care centers provide a great deal more supervised care, as well as the services described above. Adult day care is not designed for persons who are bedridden, severely disoriented, or potentially harmful or disruptive.

Adult day care centers are usually reasonably priced, but are seldom compensated by third party payers such as insurance companies or government agencies.

CASE #12

Ellen and Harry are both in their eighties, and mentally and physically healthy. They live together in a home which they own free and clear. Although they managed to save some money, an illness several years ago depleted their funds. Without savings interest to supplement their small retirement income and Social Security, they are having a difficult time maintaining the upkeep on their home and paying for property taxes which seem to go up every year. They do not want to ask for support from their children and wouldn't accept it if it were offered. They are afraid that they will lose their home because they can't keep up these payments.

Ellen and Harry have some interesting options which have recently become available in some parts of the country. These come under the general heading of *home equity conversions*. For most older persons, their greatest asset is the home they own. They may be sitting on $30,000 to $100,000 worth of assets but are not able to use that money to meet their living expenses. In fact, the increasing value of one's home may actually work against the older person, because property taxes increase, and on a set income it may become increasingly difficult to pay those taxes.

Home equity conversions allow the elderly homeowner to gain access to her home-bound assets. This can be done in one of two ways. The first way involves selling your home to a lending agency such as a bank or savings and loan, with an immediate lease-back arrangement. This agreement allows the person to continue living in the house but the house no longer belongs to her. At the time that the homeowner sells the home, a lease is also signed which specifies that the former homeowner can continue to live in the house for a specified time, usually for the remainder of her lifetime. In return the former owner, now renter, agrees to pay a specified amount of rent.

The obvious disadvantages of this arrangement are that the elderly person no longer owns her home and has to pay rent. On the other hand, she now has access to the money which was tied up in her home and is no longer responsible for its upkeep or property taxes.

The other approach to home equity conversions involves essentially using the home as collateral to obtain a loan. In this case the "loan" is a series of monthly payments which is provided to you by a lending institution. The loan payback provisions vary but basically, if and when the home is sold, the lender is entitled to all money required to repay the loan. Remaining funds could then go to the former homeowner's estate.

These home equity conversions provide interesting possibilities for older persons who are land-rich but money-poor and in jeopardy of losing their homes. But they are certainly not without risks and naturally need to be pursued with great caution and good legal advice.

All of the services discussed in this chapter fill special needs, but unfortunately they are not available in all communities. Even if they are available they may be difficult to locate. The phone book is a good place to start. Listings for nursing homes and home health care agencies often describe which services they provide. Hospital social service departments can help in finding desired services. Many larger towns also have councils on aging which oversee public programs for the elderly. These councils should be able to provide advice concerning available options. If there is no council in your town, the council at the nearest larger town should be able to provide information for your area. Finally if there is a college or university in your town, a call to the social work, sociology, or psychology department might be helpful.

CHAPTER 3

The Nursing Home: An Overview

In this chapter we will take a general look at the institution called a nursing home. Actually the term nursing home is not a terribly useful one, because people use it to describe so many different kinds of institutions, many of which bear little resemblance to what we will call a nursing home. Many elderly people consider any kind of housing for older persons, other than their own homes, to be nursing homes. Boarding homes, for instance, are often called nursing homes.

SOME DEFINITIONS

In this book we will use the term in a much narrower sense to describe only those housing arrangements with the special characteristics or features of a "total institution" or an institution which has a great deal of control over a person's life. Scientists who study the aging process and needs of the elderly (gerontologists) consider nursing homes to be total institutions, in part because virtually all of a resident's daily activities occur within the institution. While visitors and staff members may come and go after several hours or after working a shift, the resident always stays in the same setting.

Furthermore, much of what happens in a nursing home is determined by the staff and home's policies. In a nursing home your mother will have far less control over things that we usually take for granted, such as when to eat a meal or take a bath. It is not much of an exaggeration to say that the nursing home becomes the resident's "world" and that the resident becomes extremely dependent upon the home for her overall quality of life. This very high level of dependency upon the nursing home and its staff accounts for the extreme importance of choosing a good nursing home which will meet your mother's needs.

Depending on the level of care provided, nursing homes are

usually categorized as "intermediate care nursing homes" or "skilled care nursing homes." Intermediate care facilities provide care for the elderly who benefit from around-the-clock assistance because of debilities resulting from physical or mental changes such as periodic memory loss, confusion or general physical frailty. While they have these problems, they can still perform many of the activities of daily living such as dressing and eating without assistance. Intermediate care facilities provide supportive care with a minimum of medical care. If your mother does not require a great deal of medical care, an intermediate care facility may be more appropriate.

Skilled nursing facilities provide complex medical care, in some cases total care, for the seriously mentally or physically impaired. Skilled nursing facilities are usually more medically oriented than intermediate care homes and are the appropriate choices when recuperating from surgery or in other situations where round-the-clock medical care is required. Skilled care is more expensive, but frequently some of the cost is defrayed by insurance or Medicare. Intermediate level care is generally less expensive, but the cost is usually paid entirely by the resident. There is one notable exception to this, Medicaid, which is discussed in chapter nine.

Many nursing homes offer both types of care within the same facility. Generally, the two levels of care will be in separate parts of the building, so there will be an intermediate care wing or floor and a skilled care wing or floor.

THE SOCIAL ENVIRONMENT

Both intermediate and skilled care nursing homes offer a wide range of services. Indeed, because we are dealing with a total institution, the average nursing home must be prepared to provide *all* of the social, psychological and medical services necessary to maintain an adequate lifestyle. Naturally, all of the basic needs of daily living such as bathing, dressing, eating, and physical care must be met, but in addition, the special social and psychological needs of *each individual* resident must be addressed by providing a supportive social environment. The importance of providing an adequate social environment cannot be overemphasized. Imagine yourself limited to staying in your house twenty-four hours a day, seven days a week, fifty-two weeks a year. You would be doing virtually everything in your house. That would make the environment of your home very important. When nursing homes fall short of providing good care, this social / psychological area is often where the greatest problems lie.

We have defined the nursing home as a home for older persons with special social, psychological, and physical needs. The "average" nursing home resident is female and in her late seventies or early eighties. Many are alone without close relatives, and fewer than one in ten has a living spouse. Most come to the nursing home from their homes, with only about a third coming directly from a hospital. Only about half are able to get around, and about half have some mental impairment. Over half have three or more debilitating health conditions and take an average of just over four different drugs each day. While they do serve an essentially older clientele, many nursing homes, particularly skilled nursing homes, serve a much wider population. Essentially they meet the needs of all persons, regardless of age, who are in need of long-term or rehabilitative care that is not available through home care or hospitals. While you are likely to find the largest proportion of residents to be senior citizens, a wide range of conditions and ages will be found. It is good practice, however, to separate residents by ability and age, and most good nursing homes do this.

It is essential that the nursing home provide a complete social environment, but this is not an easy task. One of the things that makes it so difficult is rooted in the variety that is found among residents. Nursing home residents range from those who need virtually total physical care to those who can manage reasonably well. They range from those who are mentally sharp to those who are confused much or most of the time. In addition many different social backgrounds and interests are represented. To meet all of these needs successfully as well as economically is a difficult goal but one to which all nursing homes must be thoroughly and continually committed.

PERSONNEL

The quality of care depends not so much on the physical facilities (although they are important) as it does on the quality of the staff that will work with your mother. Because the nursing home provides so many services, you will find many different types of people working there.

The chief administrator of the nursing home, who is usually referred to as the director administrator, has overall responsibility for the functioning of the nursing home. The administrator may be the owner of the nursing home, or may manage the nursing home for an individual or a corporation. Today, privately owned nursing homes are rapidly becoming extinct as they are bought out by nursing home corporations. The larger corporations own literally hundreds of homes. Ownership, per se, is not necessarily an issue to be concerned about. In general the quality of care is less related to whether the nursing home is privately owned or corporation owned than it is related to the attitude and knowledge of the administrator who runs a particular nursing home. Indeed, the administrator sets the tone for the entire nursing home operation. It becomes very difficult for the staff to provide quality care if the administrator's primary emphasis is on the economic aspects of nursing home care.

The better nursing homes have well-educated and dedicated administrators who are committed to providing high quality care, and who support and motivate their staff members to have the same high level of commitment. One way in which this commitment to quality care is nurtured is through educational programs where future administrators learn about the needs of the elderly. Unfortunately, in many areas it is still possible to be a nursing home administrator without having any formal knowledge about the aging process or the special needs of the elderly.

In some cases nursing homes have become so large that the chief administrator has little day-to-day contact with staff and residents. In these situations you may find an assistant administrator who handles the routine day-to-day business of running the nursing home. Often this individual is a registered nurse (RN). Registered nurses have completed a rigorous course of study at a hospital or college-based school of nursing. To be a registered nurse usually requires three to four years of post high school education. Registered nurses, in addition to handling many of the daily administrative tasks, also oversee the nursing care provided to residents.

Most nursing homes also employ a number of licensed practical nurses (LPNs). While the education of LPNs is not as extensive as that of registered nurses, they must also go through a period of formal education and are qualified to perform a variety of medical procedures under the supervision of a registered nurse.

Much of the medically oriented care received by your mother will probably be provided by an LPN.

The largest single group of employees in the nursing home consists of nurse's aides. Unlike registered nurses and licensed practical nurses, nurse's aides are not required to have any formal education and much of their training is "on the job." Some states are now beginning to recognize the folly of this arrangement and are requiring either on-the-job training programs or formal education programs prior to employment as a nurse's aide. The aides provide most of the direct patient care and within a short period of time will play a central role in your mother's life. It has been estimated that about eighty to ninety percent of the services delivered in nursing homes are delivered by nurse's aides.

The social worker in the nursing home handles many of the administrative tasks related to admitting a person and maintaining a good nursing home–family relationship after admission. Social workers are college graduates who usually have a solid background in psychology and sociology. They can be very helpful to both residents and their families before the move and later in adjusting to nursing home life. The social worker is also often the person who helps you wade through the interminable stacks of paperwork which frequently accompany the move into a nursing home.

One of the most important employees of the nursing home is the activity director who has the responsibility of organizing the social atmosphere of the nursing home so that residents find nursing home life relatively comfortable and stimulating. In the last fifteen years or so there has been a great improvement in the quality of nursing home care, and much of it has come through the recognition of the importance of the activity director. In the past, many nursing homes did not have activity directors and often relied on volunteers to provide a few hours of social stimulation a week. The result of this practice was a sterile social atmosphere which often hastened the physical and mental decline of the residents.

At the present time, trained activity directors are required virtually everywhere, although the job's standards are still not clearly defined. Many activity directors are college graduates with backgrounds in psychology, sociology, and recreational therapy. In addition to planning overall nursing home activities, activity directors also coordinate the work of nursing home volunteers who help provide many essential social services in the nursing homes.

Nursing homes also employ a number of other specialists, usually on a part-time basis. Physical therapists are college graduates who have been trained to help in the rehabilitation of persons with injuries affecting the muscles, joints, bones, and nerves. Speech therapists are college graduates who help residents overcome speech problems associated with strokes, dementia, and other diseases. Dieticians are college graduates who have specialized in meeting the nutritional needs of the elderly and are responsible for developing the specialized diets often required by nursing home residents.

Physicians generally do not play a central role in nursing homes. Most nursing homes do not have a staff physician, but do have a physician on an "on call" basis. Residents are usually free to retain their private physicians, but you should be aware that many physicians do not care to make visits to nursing homes.

Some nursing homes also employ a minister on their staffs. Many gerontologists feel that all nursing homes should have at least a part-time minister on the staff, but unfortunately this is not required by law. Many members of the clergy do include nursing homes on their visitation rounds, and this does fill the void somewhat. However, occasional visits do not provide the opportunity for the formation of supportive relationships.

THE LIVING SPACE

You will be surprised at the variety which can be found in nursing homes, especially in intermediate care nursing homes. They all have to meet minimum state requirements, but there are many options concerning style and appearance. Some may have a hospital atmosphere, while others may look more like luxury hotels.

Most nursing home rooms offer double rooms, although a few single rooms may be available. The rooms are usually situated along hallways with a nurses' station at the juncture of the hallways. Nurses' stations are frequently the center of activity in nursing homes because residents, staff, and families tend to congregate at these points.

The residents' rooms are furnished with the basics for each resident: a bed, a dresser, an easy chair, a writing desk, and closet. Many nursing homes now allow residents to bring some of their own furniture as long as it fits in the appropriate places.

In addition to the individual rooms, nursing homes also have public rooms. The number of public places will vary with the size of the nursing home, but usually there will be a large lounge area, a dining area, and a multipurpose room. Additional rooms can include specialized activity rooms, counseling rooms, visiting rooms, for residents to entertain their families and other guests, examination rooms, a library, and a chapel. In general it is more advantageous to have fewer multipurpose rooms and more rooms set aside for specific purposes, because this gives programs stronger identities and people have more opportunity to engage in a wider range of activities at all times.

The purpose of this chapter has been to provide an overview of the average nursing home. Let us now look at the nursing home in more detail by examining some of the specific things you might look for when choosing one.

CHAPTER 4

Choosing the Nursing Home

In this chapter we will look more specifically at some of the things which should be considered when choosing a nursing home. Nursing homes are definitely not alike and comparison shopping is as applicable to choosing a good nursing home as it is to choosing any other product. Some systematic looking around will help you find the home that best meets your mother's needs.

There are a number of very good reasons for doing a little shopping around. For instance, while all nursing homes must meet basic standards, the actual quality of care given varies considerably from one nursing home to another. In addition to this basic quality consideration is the consideration that nursing homes often emphasize different types of care. One nursing home may emphasize physical care while another will place more emphasis on social and psychological care. Finally, as is true for people, nursing homes have different personalities. Some are more formal while others feel like you are walking into a well-liked neighbor's home.

FINDING A NURSING HOME

Begin your search by making a list of nursing homes in your area. Usually you can get a pretty complete list from the Yellow Pages. Next get a map of your city and mark each one's location. Geographic location should play a small part in deciding which nursing homes to visit. For instance, if your mother is from a rural background she might be happier with a nursing home in the country rather than in the middle of the city. Or your mother may still have many friends living in her neighborhood, and a nursing home in that area will make it possible for them to continue to visit each other. If possible, the nursing home should be located on the regular travel pattern of the friends and relatives who are most likely to visit. This may reduce the sense of isolation your mother will probably feel when entering the nursing home, and will probably lead to more visits being made because they can be combined with other trips such as coming home from work.

As you look through the Yellow Pages to make your list of nursing homes you will probably notice that many advertise that they are state licensed. This may sound impressive but it really doesn't mean too much. In the first place, all nursing homes have to be licensed, and in the second place it only means that the nursing home meets the state requirements. These requirements usually represent minimum levels of care rather than desirable levels of care. It would be most unwise to consider a nursing home which is on a "probationary" status because it has not met the minimum standards. Nursing homes usually display their licence to operate in a prominent place. If you don't see it, ask about licensing. If you have any doubts, the state health agency in your area will be able to provide you with information.

Later in this chapter you will find a checklist designed to help you assess the various nursing homes you visit. Before you actually begin your visits, go through the checklist and add any items of importance to you. Because not all things will be equally important in all cases, it is also a good idea to mark those items which have the greatest relevance to your mother's needs.

If your mother is moving into a nursing home for recuperation from surgery and she will be moving back home shortly, medically oriented characteristics will probably be most important and your task will be reasonably simple. On the other hand, if the nursing home will be your mother's home for the rest of her life, the social and psychological aspects will assume great importance to her welfare and adjustment.

Give yourself plenty of time for each visit. The afternoons are good times for visits because therapy sessions and other routines are usually not conducted during that time. You will probably get a better idea of the overall life in the nursing home in the afternoon. Schedule your visit so that you arrive halfway through lunch or late enough to observe dinner before you leave. That way you can take a look at the food and observe if people are receiving the help they need.

By all means, call ahead to schedule an appointment for the first visit with the administrator or the social worker. Arriving unannounced will probably not give you significant additional insight into the nursing home, but it will complicate the life of the nursing home personnel. During your appointment you should be able to meet with the administrator or the administrator's assistant, the social worker, the activity director, and the resident who is the president or head of the Residents' Council.

Sometimes it is a good idea to make the initial visits to the nursing homes on your list without your mother's company. This will enable you to make more objective assessments of the nursing homes and ensure that your mother will only come into contact with the nursing homes that you feel will provide the best care.

TOURING THE POSSIBILITIES

Your personal inspection tour starts as soon as you drive onto the property. The grounds should be well kept, pleasantly landscaped, and organized in such a way that outdoor activities are encouraged. Look for shady places where your mother will be able to walk or sit.

As soon as you walk into the building put your nose to work. There should be no urine odor or strong medicinal, cleaning fluid odor. The nursing home should have a normal, fresh smell. Occasionally there may be some odor due to incontinent residents, but this should rarely be the case. If you note an offensive odor, by all means visit the nursing home at a later date to determine if this is a pattern or a one-time occurrence.

Unless you have had some prior experience with nursing homes you will probably find your initial impression pretty depressing. Some of the residents will be in wheelchairs, some will be staring blankly ahead without seeming to realize what is going on around them. Others will be wandering aimlessly. You will wonder if this is really the right place for your mother.

What is not so obvious is that in good nursing homes you have just entered a social world in which many of these people continue to play meaningful roles. The wheelchair resident may be the retired president of a local business who is now the president of the Resident's Council. The resident staring blankly ahead may have suffered a stroke and be unable to respond, but she takes in everything that goes on around her. The person wandering aimlessly may be suffering a temporary memory lapse not unlike those of your mother.

In the good nursing home, if you look a little further you will find residents getting ready for art class or just coming from a Scripture reading conducted by one of the residents. Others will be looking at the activity chart to see what is happening so they can rearrange their schedules. Some will just be sitting happily, enjoying the hustle and bustle of the nursing home, while others will be unhappy and wish they could leave. Like your own social world, the nursing home is a world with activity and inactivity.

Now let's begin our tour of the building itself. As you walk through the nursing home try to look at it through your mother's eyes. Don't expect the nursing home to look like a private residence; after all, the diverse needs of many residents must be met as efficiently as possible. However, efficiency and comfort are not mutually exclusive, and many nursing homes do have very pleasant decorating schemes.

There are some general things you should look for as your guide takes you through the nursing home. The first of these is the degree to which the residents' privacy is respected. Did your guide knock on the door before entering an occupied room? Did your guide know the resident by name and were you introduced?

A second general thing to look for is the appearance of the residents. If you are visiting in the afternoon the vast majority of the ambulatory residents should be neatly dressed and groomed.

Finally, there should be activity. Residents should be walking around, sitting in lounges reading or talking with each other or with staff members. If no one is visible or if everybody is sitting together in a large group with no apparent activity going on there is cause for concern.

Some features of the nursing home deserve special attention. The hallways and rooms should be well lighted. Because older persons require more light than younger persons, the nursing home should appear quite bright to you. Hallways and bathrooms should have handrails to aid those persons who have balance problems. Floor surfaces should be very flat. Surface differences of as little as a quarter of an inch can send an older person on a nasty tumble.

The public rooms, such as lounges and activity rooms, should be centrally located to encourage their use. If your mother has to walk a long way to get to the lounge, she is far less likely to use it. The lounges should be comfortably furnished with the needs of older persons in mind. For instance, low sofas and chairs are not likely to be used when they are too difficult to get into and out of. There should be plenty of space between the pieces of furniture so that residents with walkers and wheelchairs can also use these rooms. Even though your mother might not require one of these at the present time she may need them in the future.

The furniture should be arranged in such a way that conversation between small groups of residents is encouraged. Rooms where all the seats are arranged around the walls do not encourage conversation and interaction. In the afternoon, the lounges should be used by some of the residents. If they are empty, try to find out why. Look around for places where you would feel comfortable sitting with your mother on your visits. You may find that visiting with her in her room does not afford you enough privacy, since she will have a roommate, and you will want to have some other place to sit during your visits. Some nursing homes have separate visiting rooms.

Another public room that is particularly important in any nursing home is the dining room. Mealtimes assume extraordinary importance for most nursing home residents. In fact, they often become *the* social event of the day. Because the mealtimes are so important the dining facilities should have a congenial atmosphere, much as you would find in a family restaurant. Ask whether or not residents can choose with whom they will eat meals. Weekly menus should be posted. Ask to see the menus for the past several weeks to check for variety in meals. If you have the opportunity to meet with the president of the Residents' Council, ask about the quality of the food. While not every taste can be satisfied, meals should at least be fresh, hot, and pleasantly served. If your mother needs help eating, ask about assistance and also observe whether or not residents are actually getting the needed help.

The nursing home should have a chapel. Vaulted ceilings and stained glass windows are not required, but there should be a room to which residents can go for private worship. Church services should be offered on a regular basis. These services include regular weekly worship services as well as Bible study and prayer groups.

Every nursing home should have an activity room and it should be used only for activities. An activity room which is also used for meetings or for dining will not be available enough. Even if the activity room is used solely for that purpose, check to see when residents can use the room. Ideally, they should be able to go to the activity room whenever they desire. The activity room, like all of the other public rooms, should be easily accessible.

While you are in the activity area, spend some time discussing your mother's interests with the activity director. Determine to what degree she will be able to continue to participate in those interests if she moves into the nursing home. For instance, if your mother has played the piano for most of her life it may be very important to her to be able to continue.

It is also important to determine if individual as well as group oriented activities are supported and encouraged in the nursing home. Group activities are important because they keep residents from becoming socially isolated, and even older persons who often become more introspective need this kind of stimulation. However, all of us also have needs for more individual activities such as reading.

The nursing home should also have a library area which is stocked with current newspapers, magazines, and books. Some popular magazines such as *Reader's Digest* are now available in large print editions and many books, even those currently on the bestseller list, are available in large print. In recent years many books have been transferred to audio tapes making it possible for those with extremely poor eyesight to enjoy "reading" by listening. Check to see if any of these options are available to residents.

Posted in the nursing home should be a chart with the monthly schedule of activities. This chart will give you a pretty good idea of the usual program of group activities. The chart does not have to create the impression of wall to wall activity (most nursing home residents do quite well to participate in one activity a day), but there must obviously be sufficient variety to interest your mother.

One activity that deserves special mention is the trip away from the nursing home. Gerontologists have found that resident satisfaction with nursing homes increases when the feelings of social isolation are relieved by frequent outside trips. These trips can include many things such as trips to shopping centers, local parks, movies, or ice cream parlors. These trips should be scheduled at least once a week and on a regular basis.

Other very important activities are those to which residents may invite their families. Your mother will be very proud of your presence in the nursing home during these family activities.

So far we have not said much about the individual rooms. The structural features of the room such as size and window space are fairly well controlled by regulations and are not likely to differ a great deal from nursing home to nursing home in the

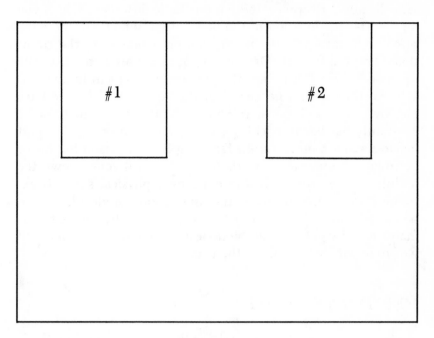

Drawing A

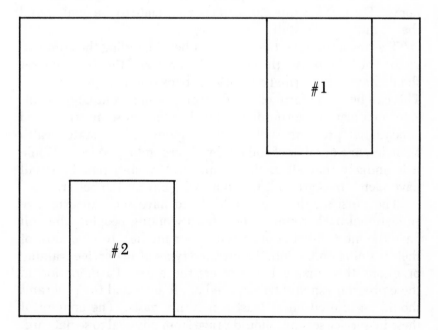

Drawing B

same locality. However, there is one basic difference which you may find — the location of the beds. Beds, which are the basic piece of furniture in the room, can be arranged in the traditional hospital format (Drawing A) or in a more humanistically oriented format (Drawing B). The arrangement in Drawing B is by far the superior because it enables each roommate to have her "own" physical space. In Drawing A the roommate in Bed 1 constantly has her physical space violated by people going past her to see the roommate. In Drawing B each person has his or her own private space and there is a "neutral zone" down the middle of the room. Having one's own physical space is extremely important and when the issue remains undecided it can be a constant source of friction between roommates. Some roommates actually put tape on the floor to define their territory, and woe to anyone who violates their space.

MEETING THE STAFF

As relevant as the physical facilities are to your mother's well-being, the staff is even more relevant. It is the staff which will control the social and physical atmosphere of the nursing home. The two key questions, of course, relate to the quality and the quantity of the staff.

The key administrative staff members including the administrator, the head nurse, the activity director, and the social worker should have some formal educational background in gerontology. This can be in the form of a college degree in gerontology, a college certificate in gerontology, involvement in some structured educational program such as those sponsored by state health agencies, or a number of college-level gerontology courses. While it is unlikely that all of the administrative staff members will have such a background, the more who have it the better.

The nurse's aides are not likely to have such an extensive educational background. These hard working people, who will have the most direct contact with your mother, receive most of their training on the job. Discuss the types of in-service training programs the nursing home offers the aides. Participation in these programs should be required of all aides and the programs should be offered on at least a monthly basis. The content of these in-service sessions should range from physical to social care. While in-service programs are essential for nurse's aides, they also help improve the work of the administrative staff by keeping their knowledge up to date. Experience is great, but one learns a lot more from experience when one has some formal preparation and knows what to look for.

Whether there is a sufficient number of staff members is difficult to determine. Certainly the staffing should comply with your state's minimum requirements, but some nursing homes do a little better than these minimums. Ask about the resident–nurse's aide ratio for all three shifts. Ask if there is a registered nurse on duty on all three shifts. Being "on call" is not the same as being there. Being on call merely means that the registered nurse is available to come to the nursing home if needed. The problem with this arrangement is that the person making the decision to call the registered nurse will have less training and knowledge than the RN, and this is particularly true if a nurse's aide will make the decision. All other things being equal, the higher the staff–resident ratio the better, since many of the problems which occur in nursing homes are thought to be due to understaffing.

Aide turnover is also a serious issue. National statistics show aide turnover at about seventy-five percent per year. Roughly this means that for every one hundred aides who are working at the beginning of the year, only twenty-five of the original staff of aides will be left at the end of the year. For lack of a better phrase, this can only be described as horrible. This has a very bad effect on the quality of service provided because much energy must be expended to train new aides and qualified aides are constantly leaving. A high turnover rate may also indicate a poor working environment and probably also a poor environment for residents. Try to determine what the home's aide turnover rate is. It is hard to say what constitutes an acceptable turnover, but generally the lower the better.

DISCUSSING THE COSTS

At some point in your visit you will have to discuss the costs of the nursing home. Unless you have some prior experience with nursing homes, be prepared to be shocked. Depending on where you live and the type of care required, the costs of nursing home care can range from $50 to $100 a day and that may not cover everything. Nursing homes generally have what is called a "basic fee." However, the amount and nature of the care covered by the basic fee varies considerably from nursing home to nursing home. For instance, some nursing homes include laundry in their basic fee while others do not. Other items such as special diets, medicine, special therapies, or physician services may not be included in the basic fee.

To compare the costs from one nursing home to another, make a list of all of the services which your mother will require, and obtain from each nursing home the total monthly charge for all services. If you are thinking about intermediate care at the present time, it is a good idea to get some idea of the costs of skilled care as well, since there is a relatively high probability that your mother will need those services sometime in the future.

As part of your discussion of finances, determine if the nursing home accepts Medicare and Medicaid. Not all nursing homes do and not all are approved to receive Medicare and Medicaid. The cost of nursing home care can quickly use up savings, so many nursing home residents ultimately come to rely on Medicaid. Medicaid is discussed in chapter nine. If the nursing home does not receive such funds your mother may be forced to leave it after her personal resources are depleted.

The checklist provided below should help you organize your thoughts as you visit the different nursing homes. When you find a nursing home you think will meet your needs, you should inquire if it has a waiting list. If it does, and some of the better nursing homes will, be sure to put your mother's name on the list. Ask if you incur some obligation by doing this, but generally this is not the case. If your mother's name comes to the top of the list and for some reason she decides not to move into a nursing home at that time, most nursing homes will simply place her name at the bottom of the list and take the next name. On the other hand, having her name on the list will greatly enhance her chances of getting into the nursing home.

Once you have narrowed the choices to three or four good homes, discuss them with your mother and make appointments for her to visit them with you. Don't limit yourself too much because a particular home may not have a vacancy when you are ready. Besides, having a number of homes from which to choose will increase your mother's sense of control.

CHECKLIST

FACILITIES		Good	RATING Adequate	Poor
1. Overall appearance of the home	Home #1	☐	☐	☐
	Home #2	☐	☐	☐
2. Overall appearance of the grounds	Home #1	☐	☐	☐
	Home #2	☐	☐	☐
3. Protected, shady areas, walkways	Home #1	☐	☐	☐
	Home #2	☐	☐	☐
4. Overall cleanliness of the home	Home #1	☐	☐	☐
	Home #2	☐	☐	☐
5. Quality of air (odors, etc.)	Home #1	☐	☐	☐
	Home #2	☐	☐	☐
6. Appearance of residents (dressed, groomed, etc.)	Home #1	☐	☐	☐
	Home #2	☐	☐	☐
7. Overall evaluation of dining area	Home #1	☐	☐	☐
	Home #2	☐	☐	☐
8. Overall evaluation of lounge area	Home #1	☐	☐	☐
	Home #2	☐	☐	☐
9. Places where you can visit with your mother	Home #1	☐	☐	☐
	Home #2	☐	☐	☐
10. Overall evaluation of the chapel	Home #1	☐	☐	☐
	Home #2	☐	☐	☐
11. Overall evaluation of activity room	Home #1	☐	☐	☐
	Home #2	☐	☐	☐
12. Overall evaluation of library	Home #1	☐	☐	☐
	Home #2	☐	☐	☐
13. Overall evaluation of individual rooms	Home #1	☐	☐	☐
	Home #2	☐	☐	☐

SERVICES		RATING		
		Good	Adequate	Poor
14. Quality of meals	Home #1	☐	☐	☐
	Home #2	☐	☐	☐
15. Variety of meals	Home #1	☐	☐	☐
	Home #2	☐	☐	☐
16. Availability of special diets	Home #1	☐	☐	☐
	Home #2	☐	☐	☐
17. Sufficient time allowed to eat meals	Home #1	☐	☐	☐
	Home #2	☐	☐	☐
18. Help for those who need assistance eating	Home #1	☐	☐	☐
	Home #2	☐	☐	☐
19. Choice of company at meals	Home #1	☐	☐	☐
	Home #2	☐	☐	☐
20. Availability of special therapy programs	Home #1	☐	☐	☐
	Home #2	☐	☐	☐
21. Availability of barbers and beauticians	Home #1	☐	☐	☐
	Home #2	☐	☐	☐
22. Opportunity to participate in favorite activities	Home #1	☐	☐	☐
	Home #2	☐	☐	☐
23. Activity schedule complete enough to provide social stimulation	Home #1	☐	☐	☐
	Home #2	☐	☐	☐
24. Availability of family oriented activities	Home #1	☐	☐	☐
	Home #2	☐	☐	☐
25. Availability of community based activities	Home #1	☐	☐	☐
	Home #2	☐	☐	☐
26. Availability of activity rooms during the day	Home #1	☐	☐	☐
	Home #2	☐	☐	☐
27. Mix between opportunities for individual and group activities	Home #1	☐	☐	☐
	Home #2	☐	☐	☐
28. Availability of religious services	Home #1	☐	☐	☐
	Home #2	☐	☐	☐

		RATING		
GENERAL CONSIDERATIONS		Good	Adequate	Poor
29. Extent to which privacy of residents is respected	Home #1 Home #2	☐ ☐	☐ ☐	☐ ☐
30. Convenience of home to visitors	Home #1 Home #2	☐ ☐	☐ ☐	☐ ☐
31. Extent to which residents are treated with respect	Home #1 Home #2	☐ ☐	☐ ☐	☐ ☐
32. Extent to which residents may bring their own possessions	Home #1 Home #2	☐ ☐	☐ ☐	☐ ☐
33. Extent to which personality of home fits your mother's personality	Home #1 Home #2	☐ ☐	☐ ☐	☐ ☐
34. Extent to which home will meet your mother's expectations	Home #1 Home #2	☐ ☐	☐ ☐	☐ ☐
35. Adequacy of in-service training programs for nurse's aides	Home #1 Home #2	☐ ☐	☐ ☐	☐ ☐
36. Adequacy of in-service training programs for other staff members	Home #1 Home #2	☐ ☐	☐ ☐	☐ ☐
37. Nurse's aide yearly turnover	Home #1 Home #2	☐ ☐	☐ ☐	☐ ☐
38. Other staff yearly turnover	Home #1 Home #2	☐ ☐	☐ ☐	☐ ☐
39. Administrator's gerontological background	Home #1 Home #2	☐ ☐	☐ ☐	☐ ☐

OTHER ITEMS OF PARTICULAR *IMPORTANCE TO YOU*		*RATING*	
	Good	Adequate	Poor

40. _____
_____

	Good	Adequate	Poor
Home #1	☐	☐	☐
Home #2	☐	☐	☐

41. _____
_____

	Good	Adequate	Poor
Home #1	☐	☐	☐
Home #2	☐	☐	☐

42. _____
_____

	Good	Adequate	Poor
Home #1	☐	☐	☐
Home #2	☐	☐	☐

43. _____
_____

	Good	Adequate	Poor
Home #1	☐	☐	☐
Home #2	☐	☐	☐

44. _____
_____

	Good	Adequate	Poor
Home #1	☐	☐	☐
Home #2	☐	☐	☐

45. _____
_____

	Good	Adequate	Poor
Home #1	☐	☐	☐
Home #2	☐	☐	☐

46. _____
_____

	Good	Adequate	Poor
Home #1	☐	☐	☐
Home #2	☐	☐	☐

47. _____
_____

	Good	Adequate	Poor
Home #1	☐	☐	☐
Home #2	☐	☐	☐

48. _____
_____

	Good	Adequate	Poor
Home #1	☐	☐	☐
Home #2	☐	☐	☐

49. _____
_____

	Good	Adequate	Poor
Home #1	☐	☐	☐
Home #2	☐	☐	☐

50. _____
_____

	Good	Adequate	Poor
Home #1	☐	☐	☐
Home #2	☐	☐	☐

NOTE: A tear-out copy of this Checklist is provided starting on page 123.

CHAPTER 5

The Entry Interview

Now that you and your mother have decided upon the nursing home which best meets her needs, it is appropriate to sit down with the nursing home personnel and discuss the particulars. If at all possible, the entry interview should occur before the resident actually moves in; however, in emergency situations it may occur at the time of the move. The entry interview is mainly an information gathering session, and coming to the interview prepared may save you the time and bother of a second interview.

It is a good idea to write down both your questions and any pertinent information which you hear during the interview, because a lot of topics will be covered and it may be difficult to recall all of the information later.

The staff member with whom you meet will probably be either the social worker, the admissions coordinator, or the director of resident services. In all likelihood you will have met this person on your earlier inspection visits. This individual will remain a key figure during your mother's entire stay because this employee will continue to be your primary contact in the nursing home.

Different nursing homes have slightly different procedures, but the interview will usually include another tour of the nursing home (if you desire), completion of forms, and a discussion of any concerns you and your mother may have about the placement. You should plan on at least an hour for the interview.

PERSONAL INFORMATION

Here is a list of questions which you are likely to be asked during the interview.

Background information:

1. Name
2. Social Security number

3. Medicare number
4. Present residence
5. Date of birth
6. Place of birth
7. Marital status
8. Who are the family members or friends who should be contacted in case of emergency?
9. What is the name, address and phone number of your mother's current physician?
10. Do you wish to retain that physician after nursing home placement? It is a good idea to determine if the physician will visit your mother in the nursing home.
11. Which local hospital would you prefer if the need should arise after placement?

Medical history:

12. Height
13. Weight
14. What is your mother's general physical condition?
15. What illnesses does your mother currently have? (List all of them and identify the most serious illness.)
16. What is the immediate reason that institutionalization is being considered?
17. Is your mother able to walk alone or with help from a walker or another person?
18. Has your mother been hospitalized recently? If so, where and for what reason?
19. Does your mother have any permanent physical disabilities such as those which might result from a stroke?
20. Does your mother have control over bowel and bladder functions?
21. Does your mother have any psychological disabilities such as chronic depression?
22. Are there any recurrent behavioral problems such as abusive or violent behavior, alcoholism or drug addiction?
23. Is your mother mentally alert?
24. Does your mother have any allergies?
25. Is your mother sensitive to any drugs?
26. What prescription drugs is your mother currently taking?
27. At what pharmacy does your mother purchase drugs?

28. What over-the-counter drugs does your mother currently take?
29. Does your mother have special dietary needs or preferences?

Financial considerations:

30. What is your mother's monthly income from pensions?
31. What is your mother's monthly income from savings?
32. What is your mother's monthly income from Social Security?
33. What are your mother's current monthly debts?
34. Does your mother own her own home?
35. What is the value of the home?
36. Does your mother have any other real estate?
37. Does your mother have any other assets such as stocks or savings?
38. Are assets available to pay for nursing home care?
39. Who is responsible for managing your mother's financial affairs?

Personal considerations:

40. What is your mother's religious background?
41. What are your mother's recreational, leisure interests?
42. What other social or psychological information would be helpful for the staff to know?

This type of information may seem a little personal and unnecessary and giving much of this information is, in fact, in most states quite voluntary. However, this information can be very useful to the staff when working with your mother, and the fact that the home is interested in this information is actually a good sign that they are interested in your mother as a person. Knowing about some of your mother's idiosyncrasies may be most helpful in avoiding misunderstandings and make it much easier to relate to your mother.

You should be prepared to discuss the funeral arrangements your mother wishes to make also. Some nursing homes request this information at this stage. From a psychological standpoint the entry interview is probably not the best time to discuss this delicate matter, but the nursing home must be prepared to see that your mother's wishes are carried out. Some nursing homes require that the body of a deceased resident be allowed to lie in state in the nursing home for at least one night so that the resident's friends in the home may pay their respects.

EXPECTATIONS AND OBLIGATIONS

The entry interview is also an excellent time to discuss the expectations you and your mother have of the nursing home. When your mother moves into the home she will have certain expectations of the kind of care she will receive. If the relationship between the staff and your mother is to be a mutually satisfying and productive one, your mother's expectations and the staff's must be reasonably similar. For instance, some residents expect the staff to wait on them hand and foot, while the nursing staff expects and encourages the residents to do as much for themselves as possible. Many potential misunderstandings can be avoided by a frank discussion at this time.

This is also the time to discuss any obligations your mother would have toward the nursing home if she decided to move out. Such a move might be necessary because sometimes, in spite of everyone's best efforts and intentions, things just don't work out. It is important to know what financial obligations, if any, you still have in such a case, particularly if your mother transfers control of any of her assets to the nursing home.

The other side of this coin is what happens if the institution should ask your mother to leave. A few nursing home residents are disruptive and because of the negative impact this may have on other residents, may be asked to leave the home. Such behavior may be entirely beyond the control of your mother, but the nursing home may simply not be staffed to handle the problem. In any case it should be determined what financial obligations, if any, are incurred in such a situation.

Finally, be prepared to make arrangements to have certain medical tests performed before your mother is admitted to the home. Chest X-rays and tuberculin tests are frequently required, as well as a complete physical examination.

The entry interview is a good time to get all of your questions out in the open and answered. Again, your mother should be involved as completely as circumstances permit. Even if all of the questions are answered in a satisfactory fashion there may still be a great many adjustment problems for you and your mother before the actual move takes place. These are discussed in the next chapter.

CHAPTER 6

Psychological Preparation

In this chapter we will explore some of the things that may occur in the time between making the decision to move into the nursing home and the actual move. In all likelihood you and your mother will not experience all of the problems discussed in this chapter, but knowing that the situations discussed do occur may help you deal with problems or perhaps avoid them altogether. The actual solutions to the problems will, of course, vary considerably from family to family. You know your mother best and you are the best judge of what should be done in a particular situation. If you are unsure of the best way to deal with a problem, advice from geriatric counselors or the social worker at the nursing home might prove helpful.

Gerontologists have long observed that certain psychological and social changes regularly occur among nursing home residents. It was assumed that these changes were entirely due to factors in the nursing home environment. While the nursing home environment does have an impact that we will discuss in chapter eight, more recent research suggests that many of these changes occur when, or soon after, the decision is made and before the person even moves into the home. This suggests that what happens during this interim period may have an important impact on ultimate adjustment to the home.

The time lapse between the decision to move and the move itself will vary considerably from family to family. If your mother has been hospitalized, only a few days may go by between the decision and the actual move. On the other hand, if there is no real medical emergency or if your chosen nursing home has a waiting list, several weeks or even months may go by before the actual move. Whether short or long, this interim period has been shown to be very important.

For some older persons, moving into a nursing home may be a very good experience. Sometimes nursing home residents have so much difficulty living at home that they look forward to the supportive atmosphere of the nursing home. Unfortunately these folks tend to be the exception rather than the rule. Moving into a nursing home frequently stirs fear in the hearts of the most courageous. And well it should. Even moving into a good nursing home requires a tremendous uprooting at a time of life when most of us have settled into comfortable routines. In addition to this basic change in lifestyle, for many the end of life is brought into a sharper focus.

PERSONALITY CHANGES

You may observe some rather drastic personality changes in your mother while she waits to move into the home. Normally cheerful persons may become apathetic and depressed. Others may exhibit downright hostile behavior toward family members and become difficult to live with. Fortunately these changes are usually temporary. During this difficult time you will have to assume most of the responsibility for keeping your relationship from deteriorating, because your mother is putting most of her energy in trying to come to grips with what is happening to her. Patience and empathetic understanding are definitely the rules of the day; it will be up to you to keep things from getting out of control. This period of life represents a major change, perhaps for many persons *the* change, in lifestyle. Many attitudes and values have to be reevaluated.

Maintaining independence is an extremely important value in our society, and the dependency which is inevitably associated with institutionalization is very destructive to the personalities of many older persons. While we allow dependence among children or individuals who are physically or mentally impaired, dependent adults are accorded a considerably lower social status than independent adults. In a very real sense, to become a dependent adult is to become a lesser person in our society. This feeling is particularly strong among the present generation of older persons whose outlook toward life was formed before government support programs were so widespread.

Dependence is a major contributor to feelings of low self-esteem in older persons. These feelings of low self-esteem generally have an impact on relationships with others. People who aren't happy with themselves are not happy with much else either. A lot of problems which would normally have been tolerated become less tolerable. If this is a problem, you can help combat this feeling through your continual support and assurance that your mother will not be less of a person by moving into the nursing home, and that she will continue to play her accustomed role in your family.

Tremendous feelings of loss pervade the thinking of potential nursing home residents. These losses range from the loss of independence and privacy to the loss of material things such as the items which they will not be able to take with them. Moving from a house in which they have lived for many years entails far more than just leaving a building. It entails leaving behind the back porch where many pleasant hours were spent with close friends and family. It means leaving behind the front yard where the children learned to ride their bicycles and the kitchen where many mealtime masterpieces were created. Leaving means leaving behind a source of memories that give meaning to your mother's life and give her a sense of accomplishment.

MOTHER'S CONCERNS

In some cases your mother's concerns may not be self-directed at all. For instance, if your father is still living, your mother may be more worried about who is going to take care of him than she is about herself. The same may be true of a sister or brother. If she is involved in organizations she may be worried about her role in these groups.

Many nursing home residents initially feel that they are being abandoned by their families. In many cases this fear arises from the popular, but erroneous, stereotype that older persons are dumped in nursing homes by their children and then forgotten. The fact that this stereotype does not reflect reality does not reduce the fear felt by many persons at a time when their whole world seems to be going haywire. This fear will probably go away when your mother has moved and sees that you are visiting or calling on a regular basis and that she is not being excluded from family affairs. Of course that doesn't help the situation right now, but continual reassurance in discussion and actions should help a little.

In addition to these more general concerns, your mother may also be concerned about more practical matters. Nursing homes are often portrayed in very negative ways. Articles relating nursing home atrocities appear regularly in newspapers. Perhaps even more influential are the television docudramas which depict all manner of nursing home abuses. These programs have had some value in that they have drawn public attention to problems that do exist in some nursing homes. However, many nursing homes provide excellent care and are not typical of the problem. However, your mother may have real concerns about physical abuse, poor food, and any number of other threats to her personal safety. Having your mother talk to the president of the Residents' Council or other residents of the home may be helpful in getting rid of some of these fears.

Other fears may be considerably less dramatic and include concerns about changes in daily routines, about meeting personal needs such as religious needs, about being around other confused persons, or concerns about personal matters such as how showers are handled. Considering the overall magnitude of the situation, some of your mother's concerns may seem rather trivial. But, as is almost always the case with us all, if it is our problem it is one of the most important problems in the world, regardless of how trivial it may appear to others. A relatively "minor" thing may have a significant impact on adjustment to the nursing home.

Often major concerns will center around the new roommate. The characteristics of the roommate are important, of course, but just the notion of having a roommate poses a significant adjustment for many persons. Most prospective nursing home residents have lived by themselves for a number of years and have become very accustomed to this lifestyle. The very idea of living with a stranger, and in the same room yet, does not sound very attractive. If you can afford it, a private room is one answer to this predicament, but few families have this option.

You might consider having your mother meet her prospective roommate before she actually moves in. If possible, arrange the meeting on neutral ground and around some activity. A meal at the nursing home should work well for this. The social worker or head nurse should help you arrange such a meeting if you think it is a good idea.

Some of the fears of moving into a nursing home are not unlike those confronting any new situation. Not knowing how to behave in a new situation can create a great deal of anxiety. This problem is magnified many times in the nursing home where your mother will have a new set of rules to deal with and will come into contact with many people who have disabilities. How will she relate to these people? What if she makes a mistake and makes a fool of herself? Discussing some of the rules and routines of the home shortly before moving in can also make the transition to the home a little easier. Your mother may be reluctant to do so, but encourage her to discuss these concerns with the social worker and the residents she might meet as part of the normal intake process.

When talking to your mother about moving into the nursing home, encourage her to be specific about her concerns, and don't trivialize them. Once she has mentioned a particular problem, deal with it in a constructive way. If she is concerned about leaving possessions behind, sit down with her and come up with a list of things which she can take, and help her to find agreeable ways of distributing other cherished items. If at all possible and appropriate, involve her in as many decisions as you can. If she is not able for one reason or another to make decisions, explain your decisions to her. Above all, don't put her in the position of being a passive recipient. Sitting down and talking about concerns will not only solve problems, but may also reduce the feelings of abandonment and rejection on your mother's part. It will probably also help in your mother's ultimate adjustment to the nursing home after she moves in. Studies of the adjustment of persons to nursing home life suggest that it is better when the resident is actively involved in the process leading up to the move.

YOUR CONCERNS

Now that we have discussed some problems which your mother might be experiencing, let's take a look at some problems which you might be experiencing. Probably the most prevalent feeling among the families of nursing home residents is the feeling of guilt. The more we care about a person and really want to do what is right, the more guilt we are likely to feel over nursing home placement.

These feelings of guilt come from many sources. First of all, popular stereotypes of nursing homes do a great deal to contribute to them. For many people the image of the nursing home is still one of a place filled with degenerating old people who sit in an abusive environment and wait for death to come knocking. Who wouldn't feel guilty about encouraging a loved family member to move into such an environment? From your own experiences

in choosing the home you know that the stereotype is not accurate, but it is still hard to get rid of the effects of the cultural
conditioning to which we have all been subjected.

Nursing homes *are* often depressing places to the casual observer. In part, this is probably because they remind us of our
own mortality and give us a glimpse into a future that we would
rather not see. However, nursing homes, in and of themselves,
are somewhat depressing and that fact might as well be faced.
At the same time, we must also face the fact that they perform
the vital function of taking care of those elderly who can no
longer care for themselves and that the quality of life for nursing
home residents would be seriously lowered in many cases without nursing home care.

Nursing homes are also depressing to occasional visitors because they only see the surface of what goes on in a nursing home.
They see only the tip of the iceberg. The casual observer sees
many older and ill persons who appear to wander about aimlessly and without purpose in life. What the casual observer does
not see is the community that develops in virtually all nursing
homes. In good nursing homes residents do not sit around and
wait for death to come. They socialize with other residents.
They take part in the activities offered by the home. They play
a role in their nursing home community by being on the resident
council and other planning groups. They help other residents
who are in need of comfort. Certainly they might do less than
they did in their earlier lives, but that would probably be the
case in any setting. For the well-adjusted nursing home resident,
life can still be very meaningful, and for many it takes on new
meaning.

Granted, most people would not choose to be in a nursing
home if they had another choice, but if nursing home care is
required, what choice is there? The good nursing home helps
people make the best of their declining physical and mental
abilities and can actually enhance the quality of life.

Another cultural custom that is a source of guilt tells us that
we should take care of our parents in our homes. This custom is
a holdover from a past when having older persons live with
family members was more prevalent. A number of things made
it more possible for this type of arrangement to exist in the past.
In the first place there were far fewer older persons to be cared
for. We have added about twenty-five years to our life expec-
tancy since 1900 when only four our of every hundred persons

were over the age of 65, as compared with twelve out of every hundred today. Secondly, in the past most persons died before the chronic illnesses that require complex nursing home care had a chance to develop. In other words, in the past older family members probably required considerably less care than do the persons who are found in nursing homes today. Today most family members simply do not have the skills necessary to properly take care of an ailing patient.

Families were also structured differently which made taking care of elderly family members more feasible. Women were far more likely to work in the home and to be available to care for elderly family members. In the past "maiden aunts," who were often called upon to take care of elderly relatives, were also in greater supply because marriage rates were lower. Because of the way our society is structured today it is often difficult, if not impossible, for families to adequately and safely take care of elderly parents in their homes. Over the years, nursing homes have developed and grown in response to a social need, but our customs have not yet caught up with the needs of our contemporary society.

The guilt which many persons feel is often fed by people around them. Your mother, if she is opposed to the nursing home move, may add to your guilt by reminding you that she took care of you and that her friend Emmy Lou is living in her daughter's house, and furthermore, if you really loved her you wouldn't put her away in a nursing home. These are tough things to hear from someone you love and for whom you are trying your hardest to get the best care available. Friends and neighbors may contribute with helpful little tidbits about nursing home disasters that they saw on TV and how they would never place their mother in a nursing home. Of course, they probably have not spent any time volunteering in a nursing home, or their mother doesn't need such care at the present time.

Even family members may contribute to your problems. Usually one person in the family ends up taking primary responsibility and if that is you, you may end up hearing things like, "Sure hate to have Mom move into a nursing home. Surely you could find a place for her at your house." They're feeling guilty too, and one way they have of handling the guilt is to dump it on you since you have assumed the tremendous responsibility for your mother's care. Of course, that doesn't help you deal with your own feelings. If you are having any of these problems, consider your situation normal. If you have avoided these problems, consider yourself very lucky.

Because of all these concerns on both your part and your mother's, the time period before the move can be quite trying for all concerned. Much of the burden of maintaining a good relationship during this time will fall on your shoulders. It will probably help you a great deal if you spend some time getting a firm handle on your own thoughts and emotions. By doing this you will be able to respond less emotionally to your mother's concerns and keep the relationship on an even keel. Sometimes talking to the social worker at the nursing home about your concerns and worries can help a great deal. Professionals such as pastors or geriatric counselors can also help you sort things out.

Talking to others who are going through the same thing can often be the best source of suggestions about how we can solve problems. Because the problems described in this chapter are so prevalent, many cities now have support groups for the families of nursing home residents. Support groups are not therapy groups. They are simply groups of people who share a similar problem such as taking care of the older person in a nursing home. In addition to getting some hints about how to solve a particular problem, these groups are places where you can get some support from others who understand your situation when such support does not come from family or friends. You should be able to find out if there is a support group in your community by calling your area's council on aging, the social service departments of local hospitals, or the nursing home which you are considering.

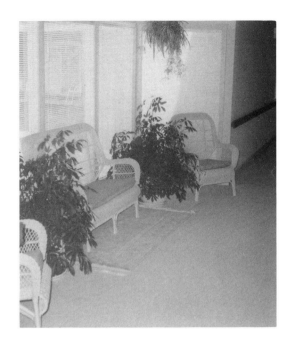

Attractive areas such as this break up the long hallways. (3)

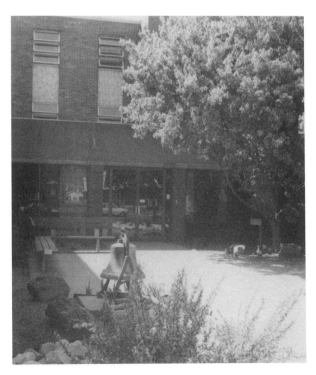

The entrance to the nursing home is inviting and non-institutional in appearance. (3)

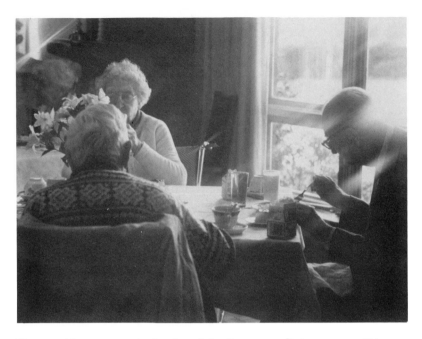

These residents are enjoying lunch in the sunny dining room. (1)

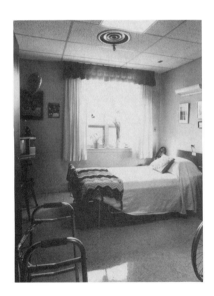 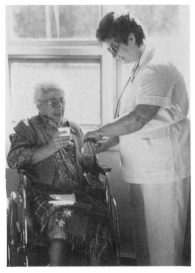

An inviting and attractive room. Note personal items such as the afghan and photographs. (1)

A staff nurse checks this resident's medical condition. (1)

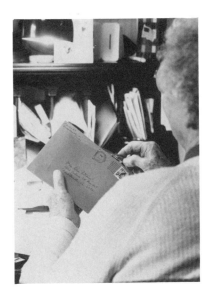

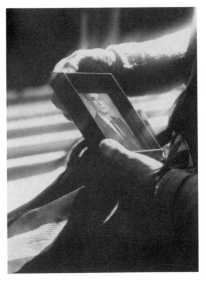

Mail provides needed contact with the world outside the nursing home. (1)

Personal items such as photographs are important to the resident's emotional well-being. (1)

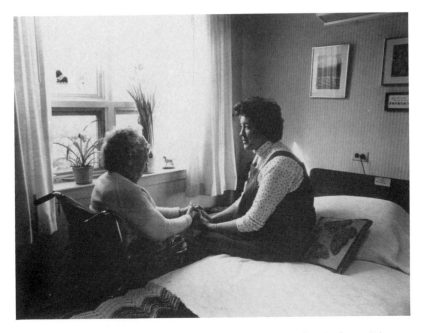

A family visitor is obviously a highlight of this resident's day. (1)

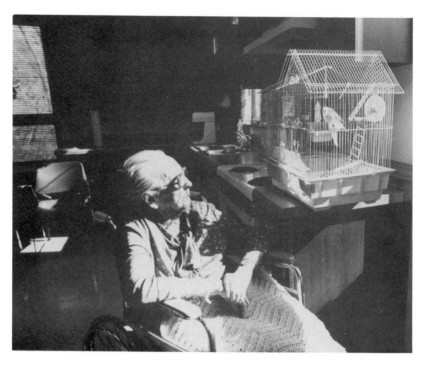

This resident is enjoying a sunny window and the company of a parakeet. (1)

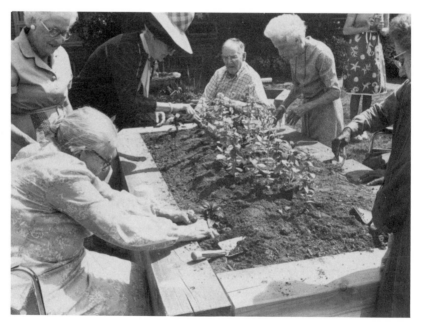

In good weather, residents are encouraged to do some gardening in the home's courtyard. (2)

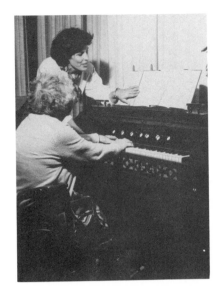

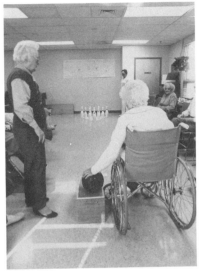

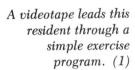

Activities should be posted for the residents. (3)

A videotape leads this resident through a simple exercise program. (1)

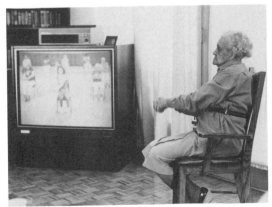

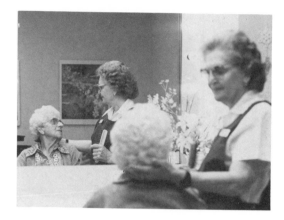

Residents are encouraged to keep up appearances with regular visits from a hairstylist. (1)

This horse and wagon proved a popular outing with residents. (3)

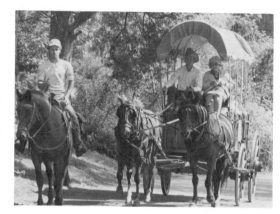

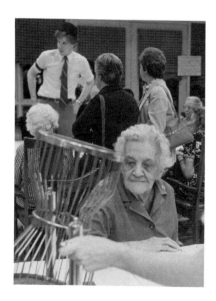

"Casino Night" at the nursing home. (3)

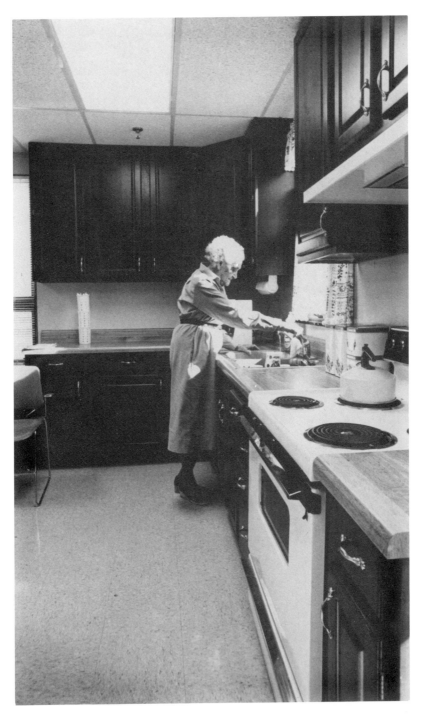

A kitchen area is available to residents wishing to prepare simple meals.
(1)

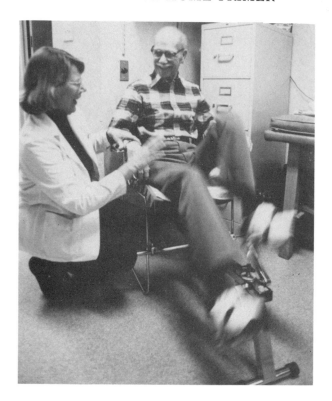

A physical therapist is working with this resident.
(1)

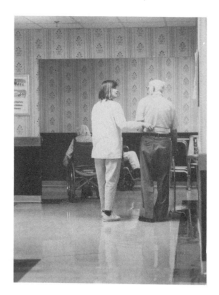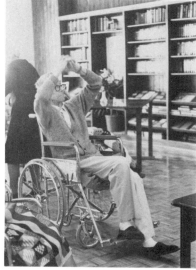

Regular exercise is very important, even for the wheelchair-bound. (1)

CHAPTER 7

Moving In

In addition to the more general psychological and social factors discussed in chapter six, there are the practical aspects of moving into a nursing home which must be considered. The major decisions relate to what your mother will take with her to the nursing home. While there are many things that go into this decision, the basic rule of thumb is not to take too much. The items that your mother will take to the nursing home with her fall roughly into three categories: furniture, personal items, and clothing. The precise nature of the items your mother will take with her is highly dependent upon the types of activities in which your mother can engage.

WHAT TO BRING

During the entry interview discuss what kinds of furniture your mother will be able to bring. Usually furniture is limited to dressers, chairs, and small tables such as night tables. Check to see if there is adequate light for reading in the rooms. If the light is inadequate you might conider bringing a good sturdy floor lamp if it is allowed. Many nursing homes allow residents to bring television sets for private viewing.

Your mother will have far more choice regarding what kinds of clothing to bring with her. The key factor here is how much drawer and closet space is available. Most of the discussion below assumes that your mother will be able to move around and participate in nursing home activities. If your mother is bedfast her medical condition will dictate what she should bring to the home with her. The social worker or the registered nurse will be able to provide you with advice. You can keep clothes that are not appropriate for the season and bring those to the nursing home when they are needed. Many nursing homes will provide a list of items and this can serve as a guide. It is also helpful if her clothes are easily washable.

Bring attractive clothes that are appropriate for the season and for the general style of clothing worn in the nursing home. Look around the nursing home on your inspection visits and note what kinds of clothing the majority of residents are wearing and bring similar kinds of clothing.

For all practical purposes, your mother will wear substantially the same type of clothing in the nursing home that she wore at home. One basic consideration, however, is that the nursing home is a very public place, so well-fitting robes and other clothing that preserve one's modesty are important. Jogging suits are often recommended for both warmth and comfort. Be sure to bring clothes that your mother can put on and take off easily without help from staff members. This will keep her from being too dependent on the staff. Your mother will probably be doing a good bit of walking, so a comfortable pair of walking shoes is very important. Likewise a comfortable pair of slippers with nonskid soles is a must.

Nursing homes have a number of special occasions throughout the year, so it is necessary to bring dressy clothes. Maintaining a neat, attractive physical appearance is highly desirable and central to maintaining a good sense of self-esteem.

Toiletry articles should include all of the items normally needed. For the safety of other residents your mother may not be allowed to leave her toiletry items in her bathroom, so she may also need a roomy and easy to carry toiletry container.

All articles should be clearly marked with your mother's name. After she moves in, check every now and then to see if your mother's name is still readable. Make a list of all the items that you have taken to the home. Give one copy to your mother, one copy to the nurse in charge, and keep one copy for yourself.

Bring personal items that will help your mother maintain a sense of identity and give the staff a sense of your mother's identity. It is very important that the staff members come to see your mother as a person and not just as a body that is filling a bed. Pictures of important life events achieve this very well. Use those frames which hold a number of pictures and change some of the pictures occasionally. The pictures make great conversation starters with both residents and staff members.

MOVING DAY

The actual day of the move will probably be quite difficult for all of you. Your mother should already have visited the nursing home and be generally familiar with the surroundings. If she has not had a chance to visit the home, the impression she gets on this day will be very important.

If the nursing home does not specify a time when you should arrive, try to find a time when there is a relatively high level of activity going on. The middle of the afternoon is generally a pretty good choice. Most nursing homes have activities in the afternoon, residents will be dressed and your arrival will be timed so that you can have dinner with your mother before you leave. If feasible, involve your mother in as many aspects of moving in as possible. At the very least she should be involved in deciding where things will be put in her part of the room.

Once your mother has moved in physically, it is time for her to move in socially. Spend some time walking around the nursing home with her. The sooner she gets the "lay of the land" the better. Visit the key rooms such as the dining room, lounge, and activity rooms and make sure she knows where these rooms are in relation to her room.

Discuss the next day's events with her and help her plan her routine for the next several days. Make sure she knows how to summon help if she should need it and who she should call for what kinds of help. As you walk around with her make it a point to meet the personnel and be sure they know who your mother is. It is a good idea to wait until the evening shift arrives before you leave and make sure that they meet your mother.

Some nursing homes have welcoming parties where the newcomers meet some of the residents. If your nursing home conducts these, be sure that one is arranged for your mother. If your nursing home does not have these little get-togethers, be sure the staff introduces your mother to some of her neighbors.

Leaving that first night will probably be very difficult. It might help to decide on your departure time even before you arrive so that both you and your mother will be prepared when you leave. You might plan your departure around an activity such as dinner or going to bed. When you leave, be sure to let the staff know so they will be on the lookout in case your mother needs something.

CHAPTER 8

Adjusting to the Nursing Home

Moving into the nursing home is one thing; adjusting to the home is quite another. In this chapter we will explore some relevant factors to this and the role that you might play. As was true with the problems discussed in chapter six, it is unlikely that you will experience all, or even most, of the problems discussed in this chapter. A wide range of situations is presented simply to alert you to problems which might occur.

If your mother is like the average nursing home resident, her adjustment to the home will proceed fairly slowly. It appears to take most residents about two months to make the initial adjustment, and it may take another ten months for the adjustment to be complete. Most nursing home residents eventually adjust, but, unfortunately, a small number never do.

THE TOTAL INSTITUTION

Before we examine some of the specific problems which you might encounter, let's take another look at the nursing home as a total institution. You may recall that this term was introduced earlier in the book. Many gerontologists feel that the "total institution's" characteristics are at the heart of many nursing home problems.

Because it is a total institution, the nursing home has a tremendous impact on the residents' social world. Physically, residents are in the home around the clock. Most regular and special events are scheduled for them; their leisure activities are largely limited by the resources of the institution; much of their lives is controlled by the staff who frequently make decisions for them. Privacy is as hard to come by as a June snowstorm.

Life in even the best of total institutions is a never-ending battle against enforced dependency, depersonalization, loss of identity, and the feeling of constantly being in a fishbowl. It should be emphasized that these things occur because of the nature of the total institution, not necessarily the quality of the staff. Good nursing homes realize the impact that total institutions can have and train their staff to deal with it effectively.

Many of your mother's frustrations will probably derive from one or more of the problems described above, but her complaints will probably not be phrased in terms of those problems. For instance, your mother might continually complain about a bossy nurse's aide. The real problem may not be a particular bossy aide, but rather that your mother is finding it very difficult to deal with enforced dependency. Finding it difficult to deal with that general, more overpowering, emotion, she expresses her feeling by complaining about the particular aide. By knowing that feelings of dependency are a major concern of nursing home residents you might be able to look below the surface and help her with the more basic problem. Of course, it is always possible that the problem really is a bossy and obnoxious aide.

YOUR JOB

Now that your mother has moved into the nursing home your job has just begun. You now have a lot more help taking care of your mother's needs, but the nursing home cannot and does not replace *you*. In fact, in many ways you are now more important than ever before because you are your mother's major link to the outside world. Many families find that personal relationships which deteriorated prior to moving into the home improve again considerably once the move is completed. Nursing homes become little communities, and there are factors which determine status in that community just as there are factors which determine our status in larger society. Children, grandchildren, other family members, and friends who visit are a very important source of status in the nursing home society.

Unfortunately, in some cases family members do not visit their institutionalized relatives as much as they should. There are many reasons for this, but unresolved guilt about having their mother move into the home is a major reason. They bury the guilt much of the time but when they go to the home to visit, that guilt wells up and has to be dealt with all over again. They deal with this by visiting less and less frequently at a time when their family member needs them more and more.

Just how much is the right amount of visiting? This will differ from relationship to relationship. If your mother lived near you before she moved into the home, you probably have already developed visiting patterns that you can adapt to the nursing home. If the move into the home was also a move to your city and you're having some problems setting up a visiting schedule, try varying the number of visits for a while and see what works out best. Keep in mind that in the first few months you will, in all likelihood, be setting a pattern of visits for the future.

Developing a consistent pattern of visiting can be very helpful because it will give your mother something to look forward to and help her in maintaining a sense of time. Because of the nature of nursing home life, residents often have difficulty remembering what day it is unless they have something to attach time to.

During the first week it may be helpful to visit a little more frequently, not only to help your mother learn the system but also to reassure her that you will be a continuing source of support and that she has not been "put away." Plan your visits so that they do not interfere with nursing home activities in which your mother might take part. As important as you are, your mother also needs to become a part of the social life in her new home. Taking your mother out of the nursing home too much during the first months can also impair adjustment to the nursing home. She may only look forward to the weekend when she can get away and not bother to meet other people in the home or participate in the activities of the home.

A NEW ROUTINE

It is important that your mother set up a routine for herself. While each resident will set up his or her own routine the following is a fairly typical day for a well-adjusted, ambulatory resident.

6:00–7:30	Rise and eat breakfast
7:30–9:00	Go back to room and wash and get dressed
9:00–10:00	Read Bible or other book
10:00–11:00	Exercise class or walk

11:00–12:00	Chapel service
12:00–1:30	Noon meal
1:30–3:00	Rest
3:00–5:00	Organized nursing home activities
5:00–6:30	Evening meal
6:30–8:30	Personal activities: read, play cards, watch TV, etc.
8:30–9:30	Get ready for bed

As you can see the schedule is full and relatively unhurried. The actual day-to-day activities will, of course, vary (see Chart 8–1), but the example above illustrates the general tone of an average day. Bedridden residents are much more dependent upon the staff for their daily routines and there is much less variation. If your mother is bedridden she will depend much more on you for social and psychological stimulation.

Visit your mother at different times and get to know the staff on all of the shifts by name. Spend a few moments talking with them every visit and show appreciation for the work they are doing. People who work in nursing homes have tough jobs and receive very little appreciation for what they do. In addition to making life more pleasant for all concerned, developing working relationships with staff members will also allow for open communication should problems arise.

During the first few weeks you can spend some of your visiting time helping your mother adjust to the routines of the home. Your mother may feel uneasy about walking around in the home by herself for a while, so walk around with her to all of the activity rooms. Doing this a number of times can be particularly useful if your mother is slightly confused or disoriented some of the time. Moving around in the home should become second nature to your mother, just as moving around her own home was when she lived there. Sometimes it takes a while for that point to be reached.

In addition to the newness of the physical surroundings there are also many new rules which must be learned. Confused residents may find this particularly difficult, and even when they know about the rule may find it hard to understand its meaning and how it applies to them.

Many residents find it difficult at first to come to grips with other impaired residents living in the home. Most seem to get used to this eventually, but at first it is difficult to deal with other confused residents who mistakenly walk into your room while you are getting dressed or the resident who kept you awake at night.

During the first few weeks after moving in, you may actually notice a decline in your mother's ability to perform even routine daily activities. One of the possible reasons for this is that moving into a new environment has made old habits less applicable and useful.

For instance, there are many things which we do each day in our own homes without even thinking about it. When you turn on the light in a room do you think about the location of the switch? When you wash your hands do you think about the location of the soap or do you just reach out where the soap is supposed to be? Do you think about the location of furniture as you move about the house? Much of our routine behavior could be described as automatic, but in a new environment everything must be learned all over again. For nursing home residents, many of whom are mentally confused or forgetful, this is a particularly difficult task. You can play an important role in helping your mother regain the ability to do the things she could do before she moved in.

The staff needs to know what things your mother is potentially capable of doing because they have no way of knowing what your mother's behavior was before she moved in. Without that knowledge they may consider her present behavior normal and act accordingly. You can provide that most important information.

Even if your mother was not opposed to moving to the nursing home, she may experience some depression following the move. If the depression does not clear up within a reasonable amount of time, discuss it with the social worker or the nurse in charge. Depression is too serious a problem to be left untreated, and the staff may not yet know your mother well enough to know what behaviors are normal.

COMPLAINTS

You may find that your mother will complain a lot during your visits. For instance, the quality of the food is a frequent source of complaints. Such complaints are to be expected. People seem to get a certain release from complaining, and few of us get exactly what we want all of the time. Also when one spends all of one's time in the same place day in and day out, one is bound to get a little testy now and then. In short, complaints will arise even in the best of homes, and your mother may become quite well adjusted to the nursing home and still have complaints.

The complaining may make some of your visits less pleasurable, but you may be the only person on whom your mother can safely vent her frustrations, and by listening you are playing a very important role.

If the complaints are about the nursing home, take them seriously. Frequently complaints will be very general such as "Nobody around here does anything for me!" Before you go off and accuse the staff of inhumane treatment, try to find out the specific cause of the statement. If it turns out that there is a problem, take your facts to the appropriate staff member and *discuss* the situation. Very little is to be gained for anyone, including your mother, by accusing the staff member of wrongdoing without trying to get all sides of the issue. In all fairness to the staff, your mother may be exaggerating the situation or she may have unrealistic expectations. On the other hand, you have every right to expect the staff to take your concerns seriously and, if there is a problem, to do something about it.

In a good nursing home the staff will be every bit as interested in resolving your mother's problem as she is. Complaints and problems are much more easily resolved if you have previously taken the time to express your appreciation for their work with your mother. This is particularly true of the hardworking aides who work closely with her. Further suggestions on ways to handle problems are presented in chapter nine.

Constantly monitor your mother's care and condition. Look for sudden changes in your mother's behavior and bring these changes to the staff's attention. By all means, participate in the regularly scheduled resident progress meetings which involve the social worker, the head nurse, the activity director, and other nursing home personnel. Listen to the comments of the aides. They work most closely with residents and often spot potential problems before other staff members. Make sure that your mother is taking her medications on schedule and be aware of any changes in medication. Determine the reason for any new prescriptions by talking to her physician. This is particularly true for drugs such as tranquilizers. Any signs of over-sedation should be dealt with immediately.

Many problems revolve around relationships with room-mates. Living with others in the close quarters of the nursing home will take quite a bit of adjustment. In the beginning things may be particularly touchy if your mother's roommate spent some time in the room alone before your mother moved in; the roommate may have come to view the entire room as her turf. She will probably resent your mother's intrusion into her space. At the very least she may feel that she has seniority rights.

Due to practical reasons residents cannot usually be given a choice of roommates, so it is possible that your mother may have to share living quarters with an individual of quite different social background and tastes. Encourage your mother to empha-size common interests rather than differences. Roommates are not necessarily friendship material; in fact, some nursing home residents prefer to keep a little social distance between them-selves and their roommates in order to retain a sense of privacy. Basically all roommates have to do is tolerate each other reason-ably well. They should not expect to become close friends, al-though it is very nice if they do.

Because of the difficulty of moving nursing home residents, every effort should be made to resolve differences between room-mates. However, if the roommate situation is really intolerable, speak to someone about a possible change of roommates in the future. Even if they are able to accommodate your desires, it may take some time for such a move to take place.

Another thing that you may notice in the first few months is an increased preoccupation with physical problems. This is a fairly frequently observed phenomenon and may be due to being around so many people with a wide variety of ailments. Physical complaints should be checked out by the nursing staff.

Some nursing home residents never seem to accept the fact that the nursing home will be their permanent home. Sometimes residents feel this way because the preadmission stage was not handled as well as it could have been. For instance, rather than leveling with the resident that the move to the nursing home was a permanent one, the resident might have been told that this was just a temporary situation and that they would be home soon. Naturally, under these circumstances the resident expects to go home.

However, some residents have trouble accepting the perma-nence of the move to the nursing home even when the preadmission stage was handled well. They just have a difficult time admitting the permanance of their situation, even to themselves. The main drawback of this attitude is that their adjustment to the nursing home may be retarded or indefinitely postponed. They go from day to day expecting to leave any moment, and never really become part of the social life of the nursing home.

Even if your mother is well adjusted, don't expect her to be cheerful every time you visit her. She will have her ups and downs just as you do. These ups and downs will now have two sources. One source, of course, is your family and your mother's continued participation in the family. The other source of ups and downs is the nursing home. Because the participation of family members in the nursing home is relatively marginal, they often don't recognize that this other world, the nursing home, also has a significant impact on the resident. For instance, the death of a nursing home friend, perhaps unknown to you, may have a very depressing effect on your mother.

VISITS

Many family members worry about what to do on visits and feel that they need to entertain the persons they are visiting. The really important consideration here is that you are visiting, not what you do while you are there. However, it does make the visits more pleasurable if there is something you can do together, and this is a problem because the possibilities are somewhat limited. One of the things that gerontologists have discovered is that satisfaction with nursing home life increases when residents are able to leave once in a while. If your mother is healthy enough to leave, and the nursing home staff thinks it is safe, you might consider taking her to a local shopping center or a restaurant every once in a while. Many nursing homes do schedule visits into the community and they are often one of the most prized nursing home activities. Since they represent a sizable endeavor on the part of the staff, the trips don't occur as frequently as many residents would like.

You are probably one of your mother's main links to the outside world and you can be a great source of information for your mother about goings on in her former neighborhood or what her friends and acquaintances are up to. You can also serve as a vehicle for your mother to keep up communication with friends and relatives.

Many gerontologists recommend keeping residents involved in the ongoing lives of their families much as they were before they moved into the home. For instance, if you asked your mother for advice about things before she moved in, continuing to do so will decrease some of the "having been put out to pasture" feeling that is common among nursing home residents. Share the good times and even some of the not-so-good times, if you feel that doing so won't produce stress that she will be unable to handle.

Actively look for things that you can do on visits. If your mother finds it difficult to write, you might spend some of your visit taking dictation for letters to friends and relatives. Many people, even adults, enjoy having someone read to them. If your mother enjoyed reading but finds it too strenuous now, get a good book and read a few chapters on each visit. Even confused residents often benefit from such activity. This is true even for elderly persons who cannot or do not respond in the conventional manner.

Perhaps one of the most frequently made assumptions is that residents who cannot or do not respond in conventional ways cannot absorb anything from their environment and therefore, do not need stimulation. Both of these assumptions are quite wrong. In the first place, people do quite frequently respond; it's just that they don't respond in the way that we expect and we don't know where to look for a response. This was brought home to me many years ago when I was visiting a nursing home and observing some residents listening to a piano being played by one of the residents. One listener appeared to be totally oblivious to the playing. There were no changes in facial expression or anything else that would have demonstrated awareness. Nothing, that is, until you looked down at her big toe which was keeping perfect time to the music. All is not what it appears.

All residents, even those who are bedfast and don't respond, should receive some mental stimulation on a regular basis. If your mother has this characteristic read magazine articles; if she is a religious person read from the Bible, play music or hymns. While you are doing all this hold her hand. It is particularly important to meet the emotional needs of residents. Even patients in the more advanced stages of Alzheimer's disease respond to emotional stimulation.

Some nursing homes are now experimenting with pets and

have found them to be very helpful in increasing communication with residents. If your mother had a small pet for which you are now caring, you might ask the nursing home if it would be all right to bring it along on some of the visits.

Many older persons enjoy watching television and it is always nice to enjoy a favorite program with someone else. On special days such as family celebrations of one kind or another, bring the family to the nursing home and celebrate there. If the home does not have a room set aside for this purpose see if you can use the dining room for several hours. If it is during the summer, have a family picnic outside on the nursing home grounds. Bring food, a TV or anything else that you would normally use in a family celebration. After the celebration take Mom home for a few hours and continue the party there. By coming to the home you are telling your mother that you accept the nursing home as her new home and that will probably help her accept it more readily. In general, encourage your mother to participate in the nursing home's sponsored activities and, if you have time, volunteer to help in some of them.

Most residents do adjust well to nursing home life. It just takes some time and support from family and friends. Your importance to the adjustment process cannot be overstated. Nursing homes, even the best of them, cannot replace family members; they only assist the family in taking care of their elderly relatives.

CHAPTER 9

Financial and Legal Considerations

In this chapter we will look at a number of practical considerations related to staying in the nursing home. We will examine Medicare and Medicaid, protective services which are sometimes used for older persons, and the steps you can take if your mother has problems in the nursing home.

MEDICARE AND MEDICAID

Nursing home care is very expensive and will probably get even more so in the future. Paying for nursing home care can rapidly drain a family's lifetime savings. Many older persons eventually come to count on one or both of the two large public health care programs, Medicare and Medicaid, to help them defray some of the costs of institutionalization.

How much support can your mother expect from Medicare in paying nursing home costs? With only about two to three cents of every Medicare dollar going to nursing home care, probably not very much. If your mother is over sixty-five she automatically qualifies for Part A of Medicare, and if she is like the vast majority of senior citizens she will also have purchased Part B for a minimal monthly charge. Part A of Medicare covers inpatient hospital care, skilled nursing care, hospice care and some home care which is not of a custodial nature. Part B primarily covers a portion of the physician's fees and outpatient care.

The Medicare Catastrophic Coverage Act of 1988 has just been passed as this book is being written. While the full ramifications are not yet clear, it appears that the Act represents significant improvements in certain areas of medical care. However, it does not appear that many of the improvements will significantly affect nursing home care.

Many requirements did not change. The nursing home in which your mother is staying must still be approved for Medicare.

Your mother's physician must certify that she needs daily skilled medical care. If she only needs skilled medical care several days a week or if she mainly requires custodial care, such as is required for many forms of dementia, she will not, in all likelihood, qualify for Medicare support.

If daily skilled medical care is required, there is one very important change in the new law. Under the old regulations hospitalization for a minimum period of three days prior to moving into the nursing home was required before Medicare would pick up nursing home costs. Under the new law prior hospitalization is not required.

Coverage for skilled nursing home care has also been significantly improved. Under the old law Medicare paid for all covered services for the first twenty days and the patient paid a significant copayment for the remainder of the 100 day benefit period. Under the new law, patients will be responsible for a low copayment for the first eight days of nursing home care and Medicaid will pick up the remaining costs for a 150 day period. Covered services appear to have remained substantially the same, including the costs of a semi-private room, meals and special diets if medically necessary, all required nursing and rehabilitation services, and certain medical supplies and appliances.

As you can see, the conditions under which nursing home care is financially supported by Medicare are very stringent and many nursing home residents do not qualify for assistance. Medicare has been criticized as being more suited to the medical needs of middle-aged persons than to the medical needs of older persons. In many respects this criticism is valid even with the new provisions.

Medicaid is a public program which also pays for health care, but it is a different kind of program and may offer more support to long term nursing home residents who require mainly intermediate or custodial care. Essentially, Medicaid is a health-oriented welfare program which is jointly run by the federal and state governments.

To qualify for Medicaid support your mother must meet certain income and asset eligibility requirements. Since each state runs its own Medicaid program, the actual nature of these requirements varies from state to state. In all states, however, the potential recipient must be able to demonstrate that she has income below the minimum set by the state and that the kind of care she needs can best be provided in either a skilled or an intermediate care nursing home.

Under certain circumstances an applicant whose income and assets are greater than the minimum levels allowed can qualify for Medicaid if she has health care related costs in excess of the allowable minimum income. This eligibility is achieved through a process called "spending down." What this means is that your mother must get her income and assets down to a low enough level to qualify for Medicaid support. Before she will be able to draw upon Medicaid funds she will be required to spend all of her assets down to a certain specified level.

Previously, this spend down stipulation was often very hard on the remaining spouse, who was usually reduced to poverty status. The Catastrophic Coverage Act of 1988 introduced some important changes in these eligibility requirements. In the past states were able to set their own limits and sometimes the allowable asset levels could be very low. The new law stipulates a much higher allowable asset level for the spouse plus a monthly income level which is based on the current poverty level and which will in most cases be in excess of what is currently allowable.

When your mother's assets have reached the minimum required level she will be able to draw on Medicaid funds. Within the requirements stated above, any monthly income she has will go toward paying for the nursing home care, with costs in excess of her income being paid by Medicaid. As a nursing home resident she will be allowed a small monthly stipend which cannot be applied to the nursing home costs. If she is single your mother may be allowed to continue in her own home, although in some states she may be required to sell the home and apply those funds to the nursing home costs if it is agreed that she will never be able to return to her home. Even if she is allowed to continue to own her home, Medicaid has a claim on the home in the amount of the medical expenditures, and this is payable at the death of the Medicaid recipient.

There are also rules which limit how your mother can dispose of her assets. In general, property must be disposed of at the fair market value or your mother may not qualify for Medicaid. Gifts to family members which reduce the amount of the assets must be given before a certain time period, varying from two to five years before applying for Medicaid. Some states allow Medicaid recipients to set aside funds for burial purposes.

In many states persons entering nursing homes and applying for Medicaid support are required to complete a screening process. The purpose of the screening process is to determine if the person really needs to be institutionalized or whether other community-based services are capable of providing the necessary care. Refusal to participate in this process may mean the person will be ineligible for Medicaid.

Many nursing home residents ultimately come to depend upon Medicaid to pay for at least some of their nursing home care. Therefore, it is a good idea to get accurate and up-to-date information about Medicaid from your local welfare department even if your mother currently has the resources to pay for her nursing home care. Some attorneys have quite a bit of experience in this area and will be aware of the most current requirements in your area. The personnel at the nursing home which you have chosen should also be able to help you in this regard, since they will be involved in filling out the necessary forms.

PROTECTIVE SERVICES

In some cases the elderly have such severe mental or physical problems that they have a great deal of difficulty managing their daily affairs. Checks bounce, bills go unpaid, funds are lost and, in general, things are in a state of disarray. When persons can no longer take care of their own affairs, families do have some legal options. The options should be pursued only with the assistance of an attorney, because they can get very complex and the details involved can vary considerably from state to state. The four basic options are guardianship, conservatorship, trusts, and power of attorney. The interpretation of these terms varies from state to state but they can be discussed in general terms.

The most far reaching of the options is guardianship. Guardianships can apply to care of a person, care of property, or both. Their basic purpose is to protect the individual from herself. Guardianships which apply to property are often called conservatorships and are discussed in more detail below.

Guardianship is a legal process in which the court places an individual, or in some cases an agency, in control of the affairs of another. To do this the court must find that the person for whom the guardianship is being established is in a state of physical or mental health that makes it impossible for him or her to carry out necessary affairs in a competent manner. Usually this means much more than just demonstrating eccentric behavior;

it involves establishing that the person is unable to manage his or her assets.

Guardianship is a very serious step which deprives individuals of their basic legal rights. In most states guardianships reduce the legal rights of individuals to those of minors. Among other things this means that individuals cannot buy or sell property or make other kinds of legal contracts, they cannot write checks, control their place of residence (particularly in regard to institutionalization), they cannot vote or drive, and they may not have control over whether or not to accept or reject medical care. In addition to these losses of legal status, there can be a tremendous loss of self-esteem associated with being declared incompetent. Many older persons who can no longer manage their affairs in a competent manner are still quite able to perceive what is happening to them and the impact can be psychologically devastating.

Because of the serious effects of guardianship, it is generally recommended that it be considered only when it is absolutely necessary and appropriate. Some critics suggest that guardianships are overused and point out that court proceedings often do not provide individuals with an opportunity to defend themselves since they are frequently not present at the court hearings.

Considerably less far reaching in its implications is conservatorship. This generally involves matters of property rather than personal matters. However, the most important differences between guardianship and conservatorship are that it is not necessary to declare a person incompetent, and that the individual for whom the conservatorship has been established retains many legal rights and protections. An individual, such as a friend, family member, or attorney, or an agency can act as a conservator. Financial institutions such as banks will often act as conservators of larger estates. These financial institutions generally charge a fee for their services, so estates usually need to be on the larger side to justify the expense involved.

The elderly person receives a great deal of protection under this arrangement because the conservator is required to discuss his actions with the older person. In addition, the conservator may be required to justify decisions and actions to the court. The conservator may even be required to assume responsibility for negative outcomes of his actions, such as assuming responsibility for replacing funds lost through inappropriate financial decisions.

Another option available to manage assets is the establishment of a trust. There are many different kinds of trusts, but basically they all involve assigning the management of one's assets to a trustee, such as a bank. Two kinds of trusts are particularly applicable to older persons. These are the "trust under will" and the "revocable living trust." Both of these trusts can provide support in managing the older person's assets while at the same time maintaining a great deal of control over those assets. Also, there is some potential for lower estate taxes.

In a "trust under will" arrangement the older person establishes a trust but controls all assets during her lifetime. Upon death, the trustee (the bank or other persons designated by the older person as executor of the trust) takes over management of the assets according to the wishes of the person who established the trust. One of the advantages of the "trust under will" is that the older person can observe how her desired arrangements are working out in practice and make desired adjustments. The older person can also stipulate at what point the trust would revert to her beneficiaries.

In the "revocable living trust" the older person assigns a trustee to manage her assets during her lifetime and declares herself as the beneficiary of the trust. While the trustee does take over management of the assets, this management is in accordance with the stipulations of the older person, who can make changes at any time. In fact, the older person can withdraw from the revocable trust at any time.

These two trusts can take the form of a custodial trust or an investment trust. With a custodial trust the trustee simply manages the assets for the older person without investing those assets. This type of arrangement would be useful for people who want to be more conservative and not risk their assets. For instance, they can have their assets in certificates of deposit which are insured, but have the trustee manage the certificates. For older persons who wish to invest their assets in more speculative ways, the investment trust would probably be more appropriate.

One of the main advantages of these trusts is that the older person retains a great deal of control over her assets while she is competent to make decisions, but even if she should become incompetent due to Alzheimer's disease, for example, the assets would still be managed according to the desires she set forth when she established the trust.

Trusts can be useful to persons who have no kin or friends to whom they would entrust their assets. Trusts are also useful to older persons who don't wish to burden their families with managing their assets or in situations where no family member wishes to assume the responsibility for estate management.

The biggest disadvantage of trusts is that there is usually a fee for the service. These fees are generally assessed on the basis of a flat fee, a percentage of the income from profits on investments, a fee based on the size of the assets being managed, or a combination of these. Because there is a fee, the assets must be large enough to draw sufficient interest and/or dividends to pay for the service costs if the older person does not wish to lose money on the arrangement. However, for some older persons the security of having their assets serviced by a reputable trustee may be sufficient to offset any financial losses. If such an arrangement appears applicable to your situation, an attorney or the trust officer at one of your local financial institutions should be able to provide you with information concerning the establishment of a trust.

The fourth option is the power of attorney option. Powers of attorney can only be entered into if the elderly person is legally able to make a contract. The activities covered by a power of attorney can range from broad to quite narrow and are specified in the agreement. The person who grants the power of attorney to another remains legally responsible for his affairs. The power of attorney can be particularly useful when the elderly person can still perform most necessary functions but has difficulty performing others such as regularly paying bills or balancing checkbooks. In this case a family member can legally be given the authority to take care of paying the monthly bills while the elderly person retains control over all other aspects of life. It is very important to specify exactly what is to be covered by the power of attorney. Everything from medical care decisions to property matters can be covered by a power of attorney, but in many states the nature of the activity must be precisely stated.

One disadvantage of the power of attorney from a protection standpoint is that it may end if your mother is judged incompetent to handle her own affairs. Thus, she may lose the protection and assistance afforded by the power of attorney at a time when she needs it the most. If older persons would like for the power of attorney to continue should they become disabled, that wish should be specified as part of the power of attorney when the original document is drafted. Often this is called a durable power of attorney.

DEALING WITH SERIOUS PROBLEMS

It is to be hoped that you will never have to confront the situation where care for your mother is so deficient that you are forced to take serious action, and it is probably fairly unlikely that this will (or could) occur in a good nursing home. Certainly complaints should be taken seriously. Too often legitimate complaints are simply dismissed as being the "delusions of a senile resident." However, it is also appropriate to look into the nature of the complaint before you take action.

It is important to substantiate the complaint by getting your mother to list specific examples of the problem or making observations of your own. If you decide that there is, indeed, a basis for the complaint, give the nursing home personnel a chance to discuss the matter with you. If you judge the matter to be a relatively minor problem, you might consider talking it over with the social worker, the floor supervisor, or even the nurse's aide and see if the two of you can come up with a solution to the problem. The quality of these conversations will be greatly enhanced if you have taken the time to talk with these people on your previous visits with your mother. If they know you and if you have shown appreciation for their work in the past they will probably be a lot more receptive when you come to them with a problem. Little is gained from unnecessarily antagonizing the nursing home personnel because, unless your mother moves out of the home, she will still have to deal with them on a daily basis. In giving the staff the opportunity to discuss the situation, you may find that the problem is a result of missed communications and that the staff is as eager to straighten things out as you are.

If you judge the problem to be serious, the administrator is probably the appropriate person to contact. Don't be concerned about contacting the administrator since he or she should be most concerned about any service problems in the home. The good nursing home director will want the nursing home to provide the best possible care and will have to deal with the consequences of any deficient care. For instance, serious deficiencies could result in losing their license, losing Medicare or Medicaid certification, or developing a bad reputation in the community, which would result in the loss of new residents.

If none of these things help but you want your mother to remain in the nursing home, you still have a number of options. Many communities have private organizations consisting of people who monitor nursing home care and help residents and families resolve their grievances. These groups may also put you in contact with a nursing home ombudsman. The ombudsman concept is a rather old concept that is used in many different settings. Ombudsmen rarely have any real legal power but, because of their position, may wield a considerable amount of informal clout. The ombudsman's role is to act as a middle man between you and the nursing home and to help you resolve your differences in the most productive way possible.

Your ultimate recourse is to file a complaint with the state agency which inspects and licenses health care facilities. Usually this is the state department of health. If this becomes necessary prepare your file very carefully. Fully describe the nature of the problem in your complaint and provide as much supporting documentation as possible. List all of the steps you have taken so far to resolve the problem. Describe specific instances of the problem and note when the incidents took place.

The nursing home you choose should provide good quality care and none of the steps discussed in this section will be necessary. However, all nursing home residents have the right to expect good quality care. These rights are detailed more specifically in the Nursing Home Bill of Rights. The Nursing Home Bill of Rights should be on display in the nursing home or distributed to all new residents. Since the actual Bill of Rights is in legalese, most nursing homes provide a version that is fit for normal interpretation. The Bill of Rights presented below is based on an actual sample from a nursing home and illustrates what such a document might contain.

RESIDENT RIGHTS

1. Visiting Hours

In order to make it convenient for family and friends, we provide open visiting hours. Family members and friends are encouraged to visit at any time, between the hours of 11 A.M. and 8 P.M., although provision for visitation can be made for your family and anyone you specifically request to visit at any time.

2. Available Service

It is our policy to provide as full a complement of services as possible to meet the needs of all residents. Treatments, ordered by the attending physician, will be provided for residents in need of physical, speech and occupational therapy, etc., provided proper reimbursement of charges is made.

3. Exercising Your Rights and Concerns

As a resident you are encouraged to exercise and express all of the enumerated rights and concerns. You will always feel confident and secure in knowing you can express your concerns without interference or threat of reprisal from the staff.

4. Plan of Care

Since your care is our primary concern, key professionals and other staff members are continually involved in developing and reviewing a plan of care appropriate for you, including treatments, results, and goals. Active participation in your plan of care is encouraged since your cooperation is essential to achieve the best possible results.

5. Medical Condition

You must be admitted under the care of a physician of your choice licensed to practice medicine in this state. Your physician and our nurses document your medical condition in your patient record. Your physician keeps you informed of your medical condition. You will always be informed of the nature and purpose of any technical procedures that are going to be performed, as well as by whom such procedures are going to be carried out. You may participate in experimental research, and there must be written acknowledgment of informed consent prior to participation in research activities.

6. Transfer, Discharge, Relocation

You are located in the facility according to the type and category of care needed. Many factors are involved in selection of the appropriate level of care, room, and roommate to meet your overall needs. From time to time you may need to relocate within the facility should your type or category of care needed alter sufficiently to warrant a change. It is also your privilege to request a relocation, room change, or facility change at any time. You and your family or sponsor will always be consulted in this decision and we will give every possible consideration to your desires, if and when relocation becomes necessary.

7. Charges, Rates, Billing and Services

A. Prior to or at the time of admission, you will be informed of our charges, rates, and billing procedure and what services they cover.

B. You will be notified at least thirty days in advance of the effective date of any changes in the rates or services that these rates cover.

C. All services provided by our staff including admission, readmission, and discharge policies are explained to you prior to or at the time of admission.

8. Personal Funds and Valuables

A. Due to the community type living conditions at ——— Center, we advise that only $1.00 be kept with the resident.

B. Should you wish to open a "Patient Account Fund" you will be provided with a quarterly accounting of your funds. During routine business office hours, and upon your request, you may have access to any records regarding your funds. Your funds will be kept separate from facility funds and upon request all or any part of your funds will be returned to you no later than fifteen calendar days from your request.

9. Grievance Procedure

If at any time you feel you are not being treated fairly or if you feel an employee has mistreated you in any way, you may take the following steps without restraint, coercion, discrimination, or reprisal.

A. Notify the Director of Nursing or the Administrator, who should be able to resolve your problem.

B. If a solution is not reached after taking this action, you may contact the owners. Such communications should be signed and the resident properly identified in order to effect the proper follow-up.

C. Your comfort, safety, health, and happiness are our concern and we hope you will give us the opportunity to assist you in any way should a problem arise. If none of the above steps resolve your problem you may take the grievance to an outside representative of your choice. The management will not discriminate or use any coercion or reprisal against a resident for taking steps to solve a problem.

10. Safety Restraint

You shall not be abused mentally or physically. You shall be free from physical restraints unless authorized in writing by a physician for a specified and limited period of time, or in an emergency to prevent injury to yourself or others, by order of a licensed or registered nurse.

A. Seclusion is not to be used as a method of restraint in this facility.

B. Mechanical restraint shall be employed only on order of a physician. A full record of restraint of resident shall be kept.

C. In extreme emergencies where immediate mechanical restraint is needed for the protection of the resident or others, mechanical restraint may be applied. A signed or counter-signed physician's order for restraint must be obtained within twenty-four hours of the time such restraint is applied. Each resident's sponsor will be notified within twenty-four hours of application of emergency restraint unless they have requested otherwise in writing.

D. Each resident under restraint shall be visited by a member of the nursing staff at least once each hour and more frequently if circumstances or the resident's condition require.

E. Restraints are not employed as punishment, for the convenience of the staff, or as a substitute for program.

F. Mechanical restraints are designed and used so as not to cause physical injury to the resident and so as to cause the least possible discomfort. Opportunity for motion and exercise shall be provided for a period of not less than ten minutes during each two hours in which restraint is employed.

G. A chemical restraint will be defined as a psychotropic drug for the purpose of restraint only, and must be given only on the specific order of a physician.

11. Medical Records

A chart is kept of Physician's Orders, Progress Notes, and Nursing Notes which is called your "Medical Record." While a resident here, your personal and medical records are kept confidential and are used only by individuals involved in your care. You may approve or refuse the release of these records to anyone outside of the facility except in the case of your transfer to another health care facility or as may be required by law or third-party payment contract. Your record can be made available to you for inspection and you may request and receive a copy of your records within a reasonable time.

12. Privacy, Association, Communication

We want to do all we can to make your stay here as pleasant as possible. With this in mind, we provide you with privacy so you may maintain dignity and individuality. Our staff provides privacy curtains when necessary during care and treatment so you are not exposed to other individuals. People not directly involved in examination or treatment of your body will not be present without your consent. Privacy is also maintained during toileting, bathing, and other activities of personal hygiene, except when assistance is needed for your safety and well-being.

Should husband and wife become residents of this facility, they may occupy the same room except when the physician indicates that it is not in the best interest of one or both persons. If proper accommodations are not possible at the time of admission, new arrangements will be made at the earliest possible date.

In special, unique, and acceptable circumstances, persons of the opposite sex, other than husband and wife, could occupy the same room.

Roommates and living assignments ("compatibilities") are important to you and to us in making your stay with us as comfortable as possible. You may communicate and visit with persons of your choice except when these visits interfere with your treatment, as indicated on your plan of care, or with the treatment of other residents.

13. Resident Councils

You have the right to form and participate in a Resident Council to discuss alleged grievances, facility operation, rights, or other problems and participate in their resolution. Participation is voluntary. During Council meetings, privacy will be afforded unless a member of the staff is invited by the Council to be present.

14. Activities

We are concerned about your happiness as well as your health, and we believe that for a person to be happy, he should have the opportunity to be involved in social and active functions. With this in mind, we maintain a paid staff, joined by volunteers from the community, who provide entertainment, games, crafts, programs, parties, religious services and many other activities. Your participation is encouraged if approved by your physician.

15. Miscellaneous

A. Mail: You receive your mail unopened on a timely basis. Assistance is provided in reading or sending of mail, if needed.

B. Services not included in your plan of care: You are not required to perform any services for the facility not included in your plan of care for therapeutic purposes and approved by your physician.

C. Telephone Service: If necessary, a staff member will assist you in making or receiving telephone calls.

D. Personal Clothing and Belongings: You are encouraged to be up and dressed as much as possible; therefore, you need personal clothing for this purpose.

The above written list of "Resident Rights" is not intended to be all inclusive or intended to take the place of a responsible, caring administrative staff and dedicated team of employees, who will always strive to provide you with love and care. After all, love and caring can never be regulated.

The bill of rights provides not only a legal but a moral and ethical basis for nursing home care. The extent to which the rights are applicable in any particular situation is, to some degree, based on the resident's ability.

CHAPTER 10

Physical Aging

A number of aging-related physical and psychological changes that may affect adjustment in the nursing home are discussed in the next two chapters. Understanding the nature of these changes can often help to understand what might otherwise be described as "odd" behaviors. Understanding the changes can also help you to communicate better with older persons. In this chapter we will focus on the physical changes.

Primarily we will examine the changes that are associated with senescence or the "normal" aging process. Senescence happens to all of us and begins relatively early in life. It is not the same as senility, which refers to certain advanced losses of mental functioning.

While the organs of our body mature at different rates, most organs are mature by the middle twenties and, broadly speaking, we can say that physical aging begins at that point. The process of senescence is an internal process (we don't catch it from anybody), and at present there is nothing we can do to slow it down. Each of us is unique in terms of how fast senescence proceeds and this variation appears to be linked, at least to some degree, to hereditary factors. A favorite answer of many gerontologists to the question "What can I do to live longer?" is "Choose your grandparents carefully." While we can do little about the aging process, maintaining good lifestyle practices such as healthy diets and regular exercise can minimize the impact of senescence.

Senescence is a very slow process and, because our bodies have such great reserve capacity, we really don't notice the impact of the changes until later in the life cycle when the reserves begin to dwindle. Then we begin to notice that things don't work quite so well as they used to. For many of us this realization first comes in the mid to late forties, and many a health spa or dieting program benefits from those of us who wish to recapture a little of that youthful energy.

While all of the physical changes we go through affect us to some degree, it is the changes in our vision, hearing, and tasting which often have the most direct effect on our behavior. These changes often occur so slowly that we are not even aware that we have impairments. Sometimes it takes a new pair of glasses for us to realize that objects really do have sharp edges, or a hearing aid for us to discover that there are sounds out there that we have been missing. As a matter of fact, most people probably don't recognize the changes until the situation gets bad enough that they cannot perform necessary daily activities.

CHANGES IN VISION

Vision is the sense that gets us through rush hour traffic or allows us to enjoy the serenity of a sunset. Because so much of the richness of life comes to us through vision, changes in the functioning of our eyes can have a profound impact on our lives. Usually noticed first is the difficulty in focusing on nearby objects or a book we are trying to read. Most persons in their early forties find that things have to be held further away in order to get a clear focus. Eventually most of us get to the point where our arms are just not long enough. This condition, called presbyopia, results from reduced lens flexibility and a weakening of the muscles which cause the lens to change shape. This situation can be remedied by wearing glasses.

The aging eye also has more difficulty in adjusting to changes in light level. Middle aged movie buffs may notice that it takes longer to adjust to the dimness of movie theaters. Long after the kids have found a place to sit, parents are still groping about in the dark. While not finding a seat is merely inconvenient, the lack of accommodation to different light levels can pose serious problems for older persons. Night driving can become difficult and uncomfortable, and moving from lighter to darker places can be hazardous. Recent studies suggest that the eyes of many persons beyond their late sixties are no longer capable of making any adjustments to light level.

Older persons often require higher light levels to see things as well as younger persons. Where possible and safe, increasing the lightbulb wattage often helps. The newer soft-light reading lamps are particularly useful since they increase light levels without causing significantly higher glare. Glare resulting from uncurtained windows, uncovered lights, or reflections from highly polished surfaces can cause real visual difficulties for many older persons.

The change in our ability to perceive colors is also a normal age-related change. Because of a slight yellowing of the lens, we may find it more difficult to distinguish between colors, particularly dark colors. For instance, your mother may have difficulty in matching dark colored articles of clothing or may have difficulty in finding a light colored light switch on a light colored wall because of this problem. Brighter, contrasting colors usually work better.

Any of these changes individually can cause problems, but the fact that they often occur together magnifies the scope of the problem considerably. Your mother may experience a considerable amount of difficulty in reading her medication or other important directions. Fortunately, devices are available which can improve vision considerably. Sometimes just putting a piece of clear yellow plastic on the printed page improves the contrast of the print and makes the page easier to read. Large print books are now available in many libraries and even current bestsellers are available in large print. A number of popular magazines also have large print editions.

Two other conditions which are generally not considered to be changes associated with normal aging but, nevertheless, are frequently found among older persons, are glaucoma and cataracts. Glaucoma is a disease of the eye which, if left untreated, will usually result in blindness. It cannot be cured at the present time, but can be controlled through medication. The test for glaucoma is easily administered and painless. Because early diagnosis is so important, older persons should be regularly tested for this disease.

Cataracts involve a clouding of the lens to the point that vision is ultimately lost. Cataracts can be surgically treated and vision is usually improved considerably. Cataract surgery has a high success record and is generally performed on an outpatient basis.

Even in nursing homes which should be equipped to deal with all of these visual changes, residents often have difficulties. It would be good to determine if your mother is experiencing any visual difficulties which would interfere with her full participation in the nursing home. Among the problems found most frequently are not enough light in reading areas of rooms and glare from windows and highly polished hallways.

HEARING LOSS

Good hearing also helps us to enjoy life to the fullest. Unfortunately, virtually all of us experience some hearing loss. There are two things relating to a sound that have an impact on how well we will hear that sound — the loudness and the frequency of the sound. Inability to discern either of these will result in impaired hearing.

Some hearing losses, particularly those related to the loudness of the sound, begin very early in life. Much of this type of loss is thought to be due to environmental factors rather than the aging process. When we are continually subjected to loud noises the mechanism of the ear may suffer some damage. When enough of this damage occurs more volume is required in order for a sound to be perceived by the ear. This type of hearing loss is often referred to as overall hearing loss. In our society we are subjected to such continually high noise levels that overall hearing loss is practically universal. The parent who tells his children to turn down the stereo before they go deaf has hit the nail right on the head. The earphones that are currently so popular are also a threat to the hearing of people who misuse them. Even though overall hearing loss is not limited to older persons, the loss may be more serious simply because they have been subjected to more noise during their lifetimes.

The second kind of hearing loss is called presbycusis. This is more directly related to the aging process. It involves the loss of the ability to hear certain frequencies of sound. The ability to hear high frequency, or high pitched sounds, is generally the most common impairment. The world sounds quite different for persons with this kind of hearing loss. Music, for instance, does not have the full range of notes and may sound flat like the old-time records sounded. More importantly, presbycusis often interferes with normal daily conversation. Different letters or groups of letters are associated with different frequencies. Letters or groups of letters with higher frequencies are simply not heard. A question like "Did you wash your hands in the sink?" might sound like "Did you wah your hand in the ink?" The hearing impaired person just hears bits and pieces of conversations and it sometimes takes a few moments for him or her to fill in the rest and figure out what you said.

Some people think that talking louder or shouting helps. With frequency hearing loss louder volume doesn't usually help much. As a matter of fact, it sometimes makes things worse. Aside from the fact that people don't generally like to be yelled at, raising the voice often raises the frequency and the person may actually hear less. Communication can usually be improved by speaking clearly and slowly. Looking directly at the person when speaking to her also helps; many senior citizens with hearing losses become very adept lip readers. Elimination of background noises is another way of enhancing communication with a hearing impaired person. An individual who can hear adequately when only one sound (your voice, for instance) is presented may have a great deal of difficulty if there is also a television or radio playing.

Another hearing problem which affects about one out of ten older persons is tinnitus. This is a constant ringing or buzzing sound in the ear. This sound is generated in the hearing system itself and the condition seems to be most troublesome at night when the environment quiets down. Tinnitus is found more frequently among older women than among older men.

Hearing loss is serious not only because of the direct effect it has on how much of our environment we perceive, but also because people frequently misinterpret hearing loss. Because persons with presbycusis sometimes take longer to respond in conversation or may even occasionally make an inappropriate response, they are thought to be slow witted or senile. This is, of course, inaccurate, but such labeling may result in the social isolation of the older person. Senior citizens may also find themselves socially isolated because others become frustrated by their inability to communicate and stop trying.

For reasons not clearly understood, paranoia, or an unfounded feeling of persecution, is often found to be associated with hearing loss among the elderly. It is theorized that this may be due to the fact that persons with hearing loss are not fully in tune with their environment and thus are constantly on the lookout for things which might pose a threat to them.

There are many causes of hearing loss among the elderly. In some cases not much can be done about the problem, but in many cases relief can be found through appropriate therapies. The therapy may be as basic as a periodic cleaning out of the ear canal by a physician. Ear wax has a tendency to harden as we age and thus clog the canal. In some cases surgery may relieve hearing loss while in other cases hearing aids may help. There have been significant advances in the manufacture of hearing aids. Not only are they smaller and almost invisible when in use, but they are much more sophisticated and can help a wider range of problems. Hearing aids do take some getting used to; it may take a month or more to learn to use them efficiently, and many persons give up on them too quickly.

Hearing loss can significantly impair your mother's adjustment to the nursing home, and it is an excellent idea to have her hearing checked by a specialist and take correct measures before she moves in. If she already has a hearing aid, be sure the batteries don't run down, particularly during the first several weeks in the home when she has a lot of things to keep track of.

There is also a decline in our ability to taste things. This is due to both the loss of taste receptors and the decreased sensitivity of those which remain. Therefore, foods have to have a stronger taste in order to be perceived by the taste receptors. Older persons often do not eat properly because eating is just not enjoyable. Some eat highly spiced foods or junk foods which have a strong taste. Often these foods have little nutritional value. Some nursing home residents complain about the blandness of nursing home food because meals must, first of all, meet nutritional requirements and many necessary foods do not have strong tastes. Also, the use of salt, which is the most frequently used spice, must usually be controlled.

Any of these physical changes can keep your mother from participating in the nursing home to her fullest extent and may cause important communication problems between your mother and the staff. Don't depend on the staff to notice these deficiencies. Many are not trained to look for them and older persons become very adept at hiding sensory problems. Since your mother will probably have to have a physical examination prior to moving into the home anyway, be sure to have the senses checked and see a specialist if necessary.

CHAPTER 11

Psychological Changes

The psychological or mental changes associated with aging are often less obvious than the physical changes, but they nevertheless can have an enormous impact on the lives of elderly persons. Psychologically based problems which are often associated with aging include depression, dementia, extreme memory loss, general personality changes, and confusion.

DEPRESSION

Depression occurs relatively frequently among the elderly in all settings, including institutions. Depression is an illness which is found in all age groups, but the elderly appear to be particularly susceptible. In the sense that it is used here, depression refers to clinical depression or deep depression lasting for weeks and perhaps even leading to suicidal behavior. It is not the kind of temporary unhappiness which we might feel for a day or so following some negative event in our lives.

Sometimes family members may view depression in an older parent as a strange mood which will go away if it is ignored. In fact, depression is a very serious illness requiring the therapeutic skills of a trained counselor, psychologist, or psychiatrist. While depression requires professional treatment, specialists can and do use information provided by relatives in planning their therapies. Most importantly, relatives often bring the depression to the attention of the therapist in the first place.

Depressed persons can display a wide range of behavioral symptoms. These include a general withdrawal of interest from things which were previously important and interesting to the person, inability to concentrate for any length of time, decreased feelings of self esteem, constant worrying, continual feelings that something terrible is going to happen any minute, and sleep disturbances. Whether sleep disturbances are symptomatic of depression is often difficult to judge, because even normally aging persons will find that their sleep patterns change substantially as they grow older. It appears that we need less sleep and that our sleep is not as deep a sleep. It is not particularly unusual for older persons to wake up several times during a night and wake up very early in the morning.

The physical symptoms of depression include lack of energy, loss of appetite, continual headaches, blurred vision, rapid heartbeat, shortness of breath, colicky pains in the bladder, chronic fatigue, stomach spasms, and frequent dizziness or fainting.

From the standpoint of diagnostic accuracy, these symptoms can also suggest a wide range of other ailments in the elderly. However, if these symptoms persist over longer periods of time and represent a sharp departure from the person's usual lifestyle and behavior, depression is certainly a possibility and the symptoms should be brought to the attention of the staff and the physician.

Depression often goes untreated in the elderly and it may well be that this lack of treatment is related to the high suicide rate among elderly persons, particularly elderly men.

ALZHEIMER'S DISEASE

In recent years we have heard a lot about dementia in general, and especially about the form of dementia called Alzheimer's disease. Dementia is a general term which is reserved for situations involving substantial impairments in mental functioning such as severe loss of memory, reasoning ability, or judgment. Dementia can be either irreversible as in the case of Alzheimer's disease or reversible as in the case of dementias related to a variety of causes including drug reactions, infections or malnutrition. Like depression, dementia must be treated by a trained therapist.

At the present time there is no way to positively diagnose Alzheimer's disease, but gerontologists are working with some promising techniques. A substantial number of psychological and physical tests are performed and if these eliminate all other possible causes, Alzheimer's disease may become the diagnosis by default. However, the only way to tell right now is through an examination of the brian tissue after the death of the patient. Because we cannot make a positive diagnosis, all dementia type situations should be considered reversible and everything should be done to try to find the cause of the symptoms.

Depression and dementia in the elderly are easily confused

because the symptoms are very similar. While this is true, there are some things about the nature, onset, or duration of the symptoms which can provide some clues to physicians and therapists. Memory loss is frequently a symptom of both dementia and depression. However, dementia patients are often unaware that they are experiencing memory loss, while depressed persons may complain mightily about their memory loss. Memory losses associated with depression may be rather mild compared to that of dementia patients whose losses will ultimately make normal daily functioning impossible. The symptoms in depressed persons usually develop quite suddenly and are often triggered by some event in their lives. The symptoms may come and go over a period of weeks. Symptoms related to irreversible dementia usually progress relatively slowly, generally get steadily worse, and last for many years. The symptoms of reversible dementia may develop very suddenly and may persist as long as the cause persists.

MEMORY LOSS

While memory loss is associated with dementia and depression, it is not at all unusual for even normally aging persons to experience some mild memory difficulties. Sometimes that name just doesn't pop into our minds at the necessary time and the keys seem to get lost more than they used to. For most people these slight memory losses are merely inconvenient and really don't have a significant impact on our lives. For some older persons memory loss becomes severe enough that they cannot continue to live independently.

The whole notion of memory is a fascinating topic and, while we have a lot of theories about how memory works, we have relatively little firm information. We do know that learning something is a multi-stage process that involves registration, storage, and recall. In the registration phase we perceive what we are going to learn through our senses. This information is then transmitted to a type of working memory which decides where the information is going to be stored. Information has to go into and out of the working memory quickly because both the capacity of the working memory and the time that the information can be held there is limited.

Information is then transmitted to the permanent memories where it is stored in phase two of the memory process. One of the "permanent memories" apparently responds more to verbal cues, while the other responds to visual cues. Discovering this last bit of information has been particularly helpful in working with persons with memory loss. A person who might not be able to respond to a verbal cue such as a name might recognize the picture of a person. We can use information like this to develop memory cues to help persons with memory loss. Suppose, for instance, that your mother is constantly calling the wrong family member because she has a difficult time matching names with phone numbers. One thing that might help is to prepare a poster that she can place by the telephone. The poster contains pictures of family members and friends with the phone numbers written on the pictures. In this case the visual cue may replace the verbal one.

When we begin to have problems with memory loss, they appear to be related to problems in the storage process more than anything else. There is relatively little loss in the ability to recall information until the more advanced stages of memory loss. This provides an explanation for the rather perplexing situation where a person can recall events that happened fifty years ago but cannot remember what happened two hours ago. In the latter situation the most recent event was simply not stored and therefore there is nothing to recall. You might compare it to taking a picture with a camera that has no film in it to record the image. A very practical problem related to this storage problem is one that family members often have when their elderly relative may not remember previous visits. Every time they visit they hear the complaint that they never visit. No amount of arguing will convince the person that you were there just two days ago. If the person is suffering from memory loss but can still discuss other things in a fairly lucid manner, it may help to buy a wall calendar and have the resident mark the calendar each time you come to visit. In future visits you can use the calendar to illustrate when you were last there.

CONFUSION

Severe memory loss combined with other psychological or physical problems can lead to what is sometimes called "confusion." This term, while not overly precise in a scientific sense, is a fairly descriptive one. Confused persons may have difficulty in recognizing people who should be familiar, finding their rooms, participating in nursing home activities and, in general, fulfilling many of the requirements of their daily affairs. Many persons in nursing homes fit into this category at least some of the time.

In more severe cases confusion may be constant, but many residents only exhibit confused behavior part of the time. In these cases confusion is most likely to result when the person's reserves of energy have been exhausted. She is most likely to be confused in the late afternoon or evening after having gone through some stressful therapy. Even pleasant events such as a birthday party may exhaust a person enough to become confused. Pick your times to discuss important things carefully so that you will find your mother at her best. It is also a good idea to limit the time that is spent on any one issue so that your mother does not become exhausted.

Dealing effectively with confused persons requires some special communications techniques. It is very important to get the confused person's attention before you proceed with your discussion. In normal daily conversation with people we assume that if we look at them and start talking to them, we will have their attention. Unfortunately, this is not always the case with confused persons who may be looking right at you but may not be tuned in to you. Asking an easily answered question will usually let you know if you have the person's attention.

Confused persons usually have a great deal of difficulty in concentrating for any length of time. The general environment in which the interaction takes place has a great deal of impact on the concentration of a confused person. The environment should be free of distracting items such as pictures or televisions. Standing in front of a window so the confused person can look beyond you and see what is happening outside will probably result in an extremely rapid loss of concentration. Standing with your back against a blank wall will be much more effective. Trying to have conversations with confused persons in lobbies or other public rooms where people are constantly coming and going may be an impossible task. Eliminating objects which may draw attention away from you will probably help, and so will eliminating background noise which can be equally distracting. A radio playing in the background or people talking in the hallway can easily distract a confused person.

If you are visiting a confused person and you are going from one setting to another such as from their room to a visiting room, allow plenty of time for your mother to adjust to her new environment. You may find it hard to get her attention while she adjusts to the physical demands (differences in light, for example) of the new environment.

When you talk with a confused person look directly at her. This will help focus her attention on you and away from possible distractions. If you look out of a window at something going on outside, you are apt to draw the disoriented person's attention to the outside, too, and you may have difficulty in re-establishing contact.

It helps to give the confused person a lot of time before repeating the statement. It may take her a minute or two to put everything together and respond. If you have to repeat something, repeat it in exactly the same way until you feel she understands what you are saying. Normally, if we have said something to someone and it is not understood, we assume that we did not make our meaning clear with the words that we used. To deal with this we rephrase our communication in a different way, hoping that the rephrasing will clarify the misunderstanding. With a confused person rephrasing will probably make things even more confusing.

Avoid making the confused person anxious or nervous, because when this happens communication usually gets worse. Arguing over something rarely helps and usually upsets the person to the point that her behavior becomes more confused. In general, it is a good idea to stay away from topics that require the use of mental or physical abilities that have been lost. This does not mean that persons should not be encouraged to do those things they still can do but perhaps just don't want to. It does mean that once an ability has definitely been lost, it will do no good to continually put the person in a position where failure is certain.

Any of the problems discussed in this chapter make adjustment to the nursing home more difficult and may interfere with complete participation in nursing home activities, even when the resident wants to participate. In all likelihood the average nursing home patient will have some of the problems discussed in this chapter. Therefore, it is essential that all residents be tested and that a complete psychological and social activity profile be developed. Without such a profile it will not be possible for the nursing home activity director to prepare a rehabilitative activity program for each resident. Such a profile should be developed not only when the resident moves in; it should be periodically updated.

CHAPTER 12

The Future

Many specific aspects of nursing home selection and adjustment have been discussed in this book. This last chapter focuses on nursing homes in a more general sense and also suggests some directions in which our society could go to improve our present system of care for the elderly. Much needs to be done if we are to meet their needs more completely than we do at present. There is an element of enlightened self-interest in this, because much of what we do in the next ten to fifteen years will determine what kind of support system awaits the present middle agers when they become senior citizens.

Most observers would agree that the quality of nursing home care has improved greatly over the last few decades. But that does not mean that we have no room for improvement. Over the years I have visited quite a few nursing homes either to give workshops, conduct research, or just visit people. During these visits I have noticed many programs and structural features of nursing homes that I thought were associated with good care. In this chapter these features have been combined into a single fictional nursing home.

AN IDEAL NURSING HOME

We might call this nursing home the "best of the best" (B&B for short). You are not likely to find a real nursing home with all of these features, but the model presented demonstrates what could be achieved if all of the good ideas could be incorporated into one setting. Chart 12–1 shows the general structure of the home.

The actual physical organization of the building is very important because space utilization studies have shown that this can have a significant impact on behavior. For instance, activity rooms are much more likely to be used if they are centrally located. Therefore, B&B is built in such a way that all of the activity rooms are centrally located in the building. The other two major sections of the building are the two wings that include the actual rooms.

Let's take a tour of B&B. As we drive up to the main entrance we note that there is a canopy (1) which goes around the drive. If this were a rainy day we would be quite grateful for this because it takes Mom a long time to get out of the car and into the wheelchair which we have to take out of the trunk.

As we walk into the main lobby we are greeted by the receptionist who, in addition to welcoming visitors, also makes sure that no confused residents wander out the front door. To our left is a small chapel (2) which is used for regular services and is open at all times for private meditation. Looking straight ahead we see the offices of the social worker (3), head nurse (4), and the administrator (5). These offices are located where both visitors and residents will have easy access.

The hallway is carpeted in very flat indoor/outdoor type carpeting. This makes for a more comfortable surface on which to walk and also cuts down on the glare which is often associated with polished floors. The outside wall to our left has large smoked glass windows so residents can see what is going on outside and the whole building has a little more of an open feel to it. As we walk down the hallway to the left (toward the intermediate wing) we pass the business office (6).

Continuing on, we come to one of the two main lounges (7). The entire front of the lounge is open, but the room has an identity separate from the hallway through the use of different colored carpeting. The room is comfortably furnished with ample open spaces for walkers and wheelchairs. The centerpiece of the room is a large built-in fish tank. Of course, it also has a large screen TV for the residents.

The next room we reach is one of the two dining areas (8). Each dining area is pleasantly furnished with tables for two to six people. Where circumstances permit, residents may choose where and with whom to sit. This particular nursing home uses a two meal a day plan with a snack substituting for the third meal. This meal pattern follows the basic eating pattern of many older persons. The work shifts and the main meals of the day are timed so that extra staffing is on hand to assist residents who need some help eating their meals.

At the rear of the dining area is a door which leads to the outside. You will notice that the central section of the home looks a lot like a donut. There is a large grassed courtyard (9) which

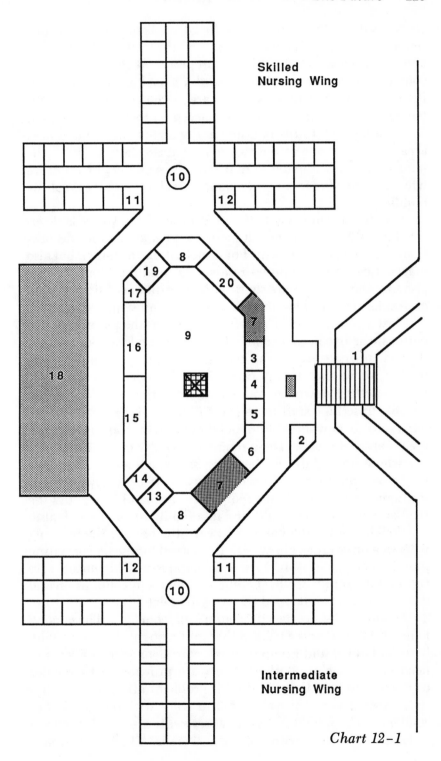

Skilled
Nursing Wing

Intermediate
Nursing Wing

Chart 12-1

gives residents the opportunity to go outside. Even confused residents can use this outside area, and the staff need not worry about anyone wandering off the property. At the center of the courtyard is a gazebo which provides a sheltered, shady area. Residents can grow flowers in this area. The activity rooms, the lounges, and the offices also have access to the courtyard area.

Coming back to the building and walking out of the dining area, we notice one of the two main nurses' stations (10). The nurses' station is situated so that the nurses on duty can observe what is happening in all of the main corridors on that side of the building.

Looking around, we notice that each of the wings is decorated in a different theme with a different color used for decoration. This not only makes the home look less institutional, but also makes it easier for confused residents to find their hall. Notice also that the hallways are short with a maximum of six rooms on each side. This also minimizes potential confusion.

Next to each door in tasteful frames are the pictures of the persons who live in that room. This makes it a lot easier for new staff members to learn who the residents are, for the residents to find rooms and, finally, for confused residents to find their rooms, cutting down on wandering into other people's rooms.

On our left is a staff room (11). Each of the two main wings has a staff room where staff members can go to relax during their breaks and eat meals. These rooms are strictly off limits to anyone who is not a staff member. Across the hall is one of the two family visiting rooms (12) which may be reserved by residents for family occasions. These rooms have a small kitchen and the kind of furniture one would find in a family room of any house.

Walking down the hallway toward the back of the building we pass a large office (13) which is reserved for use by consulting practitioners such as pastors and therapists. This encourages consultants to practice in the home. The room contains several desks so that it can be used by more than one person.

Moving along, we pass the counseling room (14). The nursing home social worker is a trained therapist who regularly schedules both individual and group counseling sessions with residents in need of such help. Staff members are provided with regular counseling to help them deal with problems affecting their patient care. The room is also used to work with the families of residents. The families of all new residents are asked to attend at least two sessions with the social worker. The first session is held before the individual moves in, to provide the family members with information concerning what to anticipate during the first weeks of residence and also to help the family members work through personal problems associated with having their relatives move into the home. The second session occurs several weeks after the resident moves in and is designed to deal with any specific problems which may have arisen. The nursing home staff work very hard to make family members feel comfortable in the nursing home environment.

The next room we come to is the main activity room (15). The room is open and staffed from 9:00 A.M. to 9:00 P.M. It is open even when organized activities are not occurring. The office of the activity directors (16) adjoins the main activity room. B&B has two activity directors and three assistant activity directors. One of the activity directors and one assistant are assigned to develop activities for the intermediate care residents, while the other director and remaining two assistants are responsible for meeting the needs of the skilled care residents. The activity director has also developed a network of volunteers to help run some of the activities. A range of activities is offered to provide residents with some choices. On the other side of the activity directors' office is a small library (17) which is kept stocked with current books in large print.

Across the hall is the area which houses most of the other tasks involved in running a nursing home such as the laundry, the kitchen, and general maintenance (18).

Continuing on, we come to a large room which is set aside for medically oriented therapy (19). Curtains can be drawn to provide privacy if more than one resident is being treated at the same time. The room we approach next is the other dining area. Beyond this is the general meeting room (20). This is one of the busiest rooms in the nursing home. It is used for resident activities which involve large numbers of residents. For instance, bingo is played here and movies are shown in this room.

The meeting room is also an important staff room. At the beginning of each week the head nurse of each shift meets with her staff to discuss problems residents might be having and to give a briefing on any new residents who are scheduled to move in that week or any residents who unexpectedly moved in the previous week. The purpose of these briefings is to introduce the residents to the staff as people rather than just occupants of rooms. The staff members are expected to be able to identify every resident by sight, regardless of which wing they work in.

Educational programs are also conducted in this room. At least once a month all of the professional staff get together for a workshop on some aspect of working with elderly institutionalized persons. They are then expected to teach this information to the aides during normal working interaction. They make extensive use of gerontologists in the area who bring the latest in the field to these sessions.

Like many homes, B&B had problems with high aide turnover. The administrator found this unacceptable from both a business and care standpoint. One "obvious" solution was to pay the aides considerably more, but she didn't have the budget to do that. She consulted with a gerontologist who gave her the results of some studies which demonstrated that pay was not a major factor in aide turnover since aides rarely have the educational background to qualify for other more highly paying jobs. However, he suggested that working conditions were important factors influencing turnover. Therefore, she developed programs to upgrade the skills of the aides and rewarded them with a bonus every time they reached a new level of knowledge. Notice of their advancement was placed in a prominent location in the nursing home. She hired an extra aide for each shift and, in turn, expected aides to spend some time during the day socializing with each resident in their area. Information from aides became an integral part of patient care conferences. In short, their contributions to nursing home care were recognized.

This meeting room is also used for family oriented programs. Regular educational programs are offered to help the families of residents better understand what their relative is experiencing. The activity director also plans at least one social event involving family members each month. It took a while for these programs to catch on but they are now well attended.

There are many other excellent features which have been implemented by innovative nursing home directors and which could have been included in B&B. A sufficient number of features has been included to make B&B somewhat unusual among the nation's 15,000-plus nursing homes. B&B places a great deal of emphasis on the social needs of the residents.

In our society, nursing homes tend to be viewed as mini hospitals. This is readily apparent from the hospital-like appearance to the regulations, which are dominated by rules specifying medical requirements in great detail while frequently only giving passing mention to the general responsibility for meeting social and psychological needs. It is not that meeting the medical needs of residents is not important, it is just that meeting the social needs is equally important. In fact, because of the chronic nature of the illnesses of most nursing home residents, there is not that much medical care which is actually dispensed in nursing homes, and much of the medical care delivered is custodial in nature.

It is the feeling of many gerontologists that if we wish to continue to improve the level of care in the nation's nursing homes even more, we need to place greater emphasis on social and psychological needs. Since state and federal regulations have a tremendous impact on what services are provided in nursing homes, setting up more precise requirements for social and psychological services would be a big step in the right direction.

Most of all we need to recognize that the label "nursing home" consists of two words, not just one. The institution is a "home" for over a million elderly persons. Let's make it more the kind of home in which we would like to live out our final years.

NATIONAL POLICY

As a society we are not stingy when it comes to spending money for support systems for the elderly. Yet many gerontologists feel that we are not meeting the needs of our elderly as well as some other countries at our socioeconomic level. Basically, we have chosen to spend our money differently from these other countries, and in so doing, we have created a system which is heavily dependent on nursing homes. While a range of alternatives was presented in chapter two, in many parts of our country the elderly have two choices, struggle along at home as best as they can or move into a nursing home.

This approach has several negative consequences. First of all, it results in the unnecessary institutionalization of perhaps a quarter of a million elderly persons. Second, it places an enormous burden on nursing homes because the range of resident needs is so broad. The wider the range of needs, the more difficult it is to meet any of them really well. Third, the approach is expremely expensive to society and individuals. This is due to the fact that many nursing home residents, by virtue of moving into the home, are buying care they really don't need simply because it is the only way to obtain the level of care they really require.

At the present time we have just under thirty million Americans aged sixty-five and over. In just over forty years that number will more than double to almost sixty-five million. More to the point, a larger proportion of the elderly will be over seventy-five and therefore in that part of the older population which requires more support services. With these demographics we simply cannot afford to maintain our present approach to meeting the needs of the elderly. We cannot afford it in human costs or in financial costs.

Chart 2-1 on page 14 presents the alternatives which can be expanded beyond their present scope. The problem is that there is little impetus to do so. Most of these alternatives cannot receive government financial support and hence go underused and underdeveloped. For example, imagine a low income family with an elderly relative who can no longer live independently. The family would like to take care of the relative, but both husband and wife work and they cannot take care of the relative during the day. They cannot afford to hire someone to stay with the relative nor can they afford to place the relative in an adult day care center (if one exists in their area). Probably their relative will end up in a nursing home and Medicaid will pay for the stay. Here we have a family that wanted to help, but our system made it difficult, if not impossible, to do so. We have a person moving into a nursing home who really does not need to and, finally, as a society we are paying a great deal more for nursing home care than we would have paid for adult day care. This does not seem like a very practical way to run things.

As a society we can pursue several options. First, and perhaps most importantly, we can support families in taking care of their elderly relatives. In an earlier chapter the myth that families dump their elderly parents was discussed, and we saw that most families take care of their elderly relatives to the very limits of their resources. Often these limits are financial. We should consider direct financial payments to families to help them take care of their relatives. Opponents of this suggestion charge that some families will abuse the program. One would be hard pressed to find any kind of program in either public service or private industry that is not abused. Medicare and Medicaid are defrauded of billions of dollars a year, but that does not mean that millions of people have not benefitted mightily from these programs. The option of support would make it possible for families to do what they really want and could save society a substantial amount of money at the same time.

We should consider providing support alternatives such as adult day care and the many supporting services listed in Chart 2–1. In the long run, we will save money if we develop the appropriate mix of nursing home care and alternative care systems. Developing and supporting the alternatives will not be enough. We also need to educate the nation's elderly population to the fact that these alternatives exist and that they can help meet their needs.

In all likelihood we need to become more specialized in our services than we are at the present time. This may involve developing specialized day care centers or specialized nursing homes where the staff is trained to deal with a particular kind of problem. Already we see a need for nursing homes to deal specifically with victims of Alzheimer's disease or other forms of dementia. This specialization will greatly improve the quality of care because the staff will be more highly qualified, as well as have the resources required to deal with special populations.

If we wish to develop a national policy such as the one suggested here, we have time. While the elderly have become much more visible in our society, the growing number of elderly persons in the next two decades will actually be the lowest in this century. We have some breathing space which we can use to develop a comprehensive support system which will both be more cost effective and do a better job of meeting the needs of the elderly. Twenty years from now we will be unable to say that we were caught by surprise. Barring any major catastrophe, we can generally predict how many older persons we will have and even what their needs will be. We need only use that knowledge.

CHECKLIST

FACILITIES		RATING		
		Good	Adequate	Poor
1. Overall appearance of the home	Home #1 Home #2	☐ ☐	☐ ☐	☐ ☐
2. Overall appearance of the grounds	Home #1 Home #2	☐ ☐	☐ ☐	☐ ☐
3. Protected, shady areas, walkways	Home #1 Home #2	☐ ☐	☐ ☐	☐ ☐
4. Overall cleanliness of the home	Home #1 Home #2	☐ ☐	☐ ☐	☐ ☐
5. Quality of air (odors, etc.)	Home #1 Home #2	☐ ☐	☐ ☐	☐ ☐
6. Appearance of residents (dressed, groomed, etc.)	Home #1 Home #2	☐ ☐	☐ ☐	☐ ☐
7. Overall evaluation of dining area	Home #1 Home #2	☐ ☐	☐ ☐	☐ ☐
8. Overall evaluation of lounge area	Home #1 Home #2	☐ ☐	☐ ☐	☐ ☐
9. Places where you can visit with your mother	Home #1 Home #2	☐ ☐	☐ ☐	☐ ☐
10. Overall evaluation of the chapel	Home #1 Home #2	☐ ☐	☐ ☐	☐ ☐
11. Overall evaluation of activity room	Home #1 Home #2	☐ ☐	☐ ☐	☐ ☐
12. Overall evaluation of library	Home #1 Home #2	☐ ☐	☐ ☐	☐ ☐
13. Overall evaluation of individual rooms	Home #1 Home #2	☐ ☐	☐ ☐	☐ ☐

SERVICES		RATING		
		Good	Adequate	Poor
14. Quality of meals	Home #1	☐	☐	☐
	Home #2	☐	☐	☐
15. Variety of meals	Home #1	☐	☐	☐
	Home #2	☐	☐	☐
16. Availability of special diets	Home #1	☐	☐	☐
	Home #2	☐	☐	☐
17. Sufficient time allowed to eat meals	Home #1	☐	☐	☐
	Home #2	☐	☐	☐
18. Help for those who need assistance eating	Home #1	☐	☐	☐
	Home #2	☐	☐	☐
19. Choice of company at meals	Home #1	☐	☐	☐
	Home #2	☐	☐	☐
20. Availability of special therapy programs	Home #1	☐	☐	☐
	Home #2	☐	☐	☐
21. Availability of barbers and beauticians	Home #1	☐	☐	☐
	Home #2	☐	☐	☐
22. Opportunity to participate in favorite activities	Home #1	☐	☐	☐
	Home #2	☐	☐	☐
23. Activity schedule complete enough to provide social stimulation	Home #1	☐	☐	☐
	Home #2	☐	☐	☐
24. Availability of family oriented activities	Home #1	☐	☐	☐
	Home #2	☐	☐	☐
25. Availability of community based activities	Home #1	☐	☐	☐
	Home #2	☐	☐	☐
26. Availability of activity rooms during the day	Home #1	☐	☐	☐
	Home #2	☐	☐	☐
27. Mix between opportunities for individual and group activities	Home #1	☐	☐	☐
	Home #2	☐	☐	☐
28. Availability of religious services	Home #1	☐	☐	☐
	Home #2	☐	☐	☐

GENERAL CONSIDERATIONS		RATING		
		Good	Adequate	Poor
29. Extent to which privacy of residents is respected	Home #1	☐	☐	☐
	Home #2	☐	☐	☐
30. Convenience of home to visitors	Home #1	☐	☐	☐
	Home #2	☐	☐	☐
31. Extent to which residents are treated with respect	Home #1	☐	☐	☐
	Home #2	☐	☐	☐
32. Extent to which residents may bring their own possessions	Home #1	☐	☐	☐
	Home #2	☐	☐	☐
33. Extent to which personality of home fits your mother's personality	Home #1	☐	☐	☐
	Home #2	☐	☐	☐
34. Extent to which home will meet your mother's expectations	Home #1	☐	☐	☐
	Home #2	☐	☐	☐
35. Adequacy of in-service training programs for nurse's aides	Home #1	☐	☐	☐
	Home #2	☐	☐	☐
36. Adequacy of in-service training programs for other staff members	Home #1	☐	☐	☐
	Home #2	☐	☐	☐
37. Nurse's aide yearly turnover	Home #1	☐	☐	☐
	Home #2	☐	☐	☐
38. Other staff yearly turnover	Home #1	☐	☐	☐
	Home #2	☐	☐	☐
39. Administrator's gerontological background	Home #1	☐	☐	☐
	Home #2	☐	☐	☐

OTHER ITEMS OF PARTICULAR
IMPORTANCE TO YOU

	Good	RATING Adequate	Poor

40. _____

	Good	Adequate	Poor
Home #1	☐	☐	☐
Home #2	☐	☐	☐

41. _____

Home #1	☐	☐	☐
Home #2	☐	☐	☐

42. _____

Home #1	☐	☐	☐
Home #2	☐	☐	☐

43. _____

Home #1	☐	☐	☐
Home #2	☐	☐	☐

44. _____

Home #1	☐	☐	☐
Home #2	☐	☐	☐

45. _____

Home #1	☐	☐	☐
Home #2	☐	☐	☐

46. _____

Home #1	☐	☐	☐
Home #2	☐	☐	☐

47. _____

Home #1	☐	☐	☐
Home #2	☐	☐	☐

48. _____

Home #1	☐	☐	☐
Home #2	☐	☐	☐

49. _____

Home #1	☐	☐	☐
Home #2	☐	☐	☐

50. _____

Home #1	☐	☐	☐
Home #2	☐	☐	☐

RESOURCES

Zarit, Orr and Zarit, *The Hidden Victims of Alzheimer's Disease.* New York University Press, 1985.

This book is written with health care professionals in mind but the general audience will still find many useful bits of information. For instance chapter three, on assessing dementia, will be particularly useful to families whose relatives are still in the diagnostic stages. The first two chapters provide the general reader with an idea of the major sources of stress and how professional counselors can provide some relief.

Robinson, *You Asked About Rheumatoid Arthritis.* Beaufort Books, Inc., 1982.

This book covers a wide range of topics relating to rheumatoid arthritis, including a discussion of the various types of rheumatoid diseases and arthritis, the symptoms and diagnosis of rheumatoid arthritis, drug and surgical treatment, acupuncture and the relationship between diet and rheumatoid arthritis. This book provides a fountain of introductory level information about rheumatoid arthritis.

Leflar and Lillie, *Cataracts.* Facts on File Publications, 1981.

The book begins with a brief introduction dealing with cataracts and their causes. Other chapters cover the benefits and risks of cataract surgery, the basic ways in which ophthalmologists deal with cataracts, and the costs of cataract surgery.

Greist and Jefferson, *Depression and Its Treatment.* American Psychiatric Press, 1984.

The book begins by providing a basic discussion of depression and the "causes" of depression. There is also brief discussion of suicide and a general discussion of the treatment of depression.

Poe and Holloway, *Drugs and the Aged.* McGraw–Hill Book Company, 1980.

In this very thorough treatment of the impact of drugs on the elderly the authors begin with a general discussion of how drugs work, the undesirable side effects of drugs, and why drugs affect older persons differently (as compared with younger persons). The remaining chapters focus on the drugs used to treat the most common disorders, including gastrointestinal, cardiovascular, mind, dementia, and movement disorders.

Alec Combs, *Hearing Loss Help.* Alpenglow Press, 1986.

Topics covered include the social and personal problems associated with hearing loss, hearing evaluations, the different types of loss, early warning signs of loss, ways of communicating with persons with hearing loss, improving the environment so that the hearing impaired can hear better, and describes assistive devices and hearing aids. While the treatment is basic, it is thorough.

Mace and Rabins, *The 36-Hour Day.* Johns Hopkins University Press, 1981.

This comprehensive book is designed specifically for families who have relatives with dementia. However, the book provides a great deal of information which would be useful to any family taking care of an older relative. Strongly recommended for all family caregivers who find themselves caring for a victim of dementia.

Mayes, *Osteoporosis: Brittle Bones and Calcium Crisis.* Pennant Books, 1986.

This thorough treatment of osteoporosis discusses the nature of the disease in sufficient detail to provide the reader with a basic understanding. The general tone is quite different from many "fad" books on this and similar topics. While much information is provided, the reader is constantly reminded that treatment should involve the advice of a qualified health care professional. Many helpful food charts are included and both the chapters on diet and exercise may motivate persons to assume more healthy lifestyles.

Pizer, Editor, *Over 55, Healthy and Alive.* Van Nostrand Reinhold Company, 1983.

This is an excellent book for the individual who desires a somewhat more sophisticated treatment of the physical changes associated with aging, but who wants to avoid textbooks and similar detailed advanced treatments.

Consumer Guide, *Your Retirement: A Complete Planning Guide.* Publications International, Ltd., 3841 West Oakton Street, Skokie, Illinois 60076.

This guide to retirement covers many of the issues which need to be considered in planning one's retirement. The importance of planning to retire, planning for financial security, making the most of Social Security and pensions, investing retirement income, planning estates and will, and obtaining appropriate insurance are among the topics discussed in this book. As a general introduction to retirement planning, this book provides much useful information.

Hess and Bahr, *What Every Family Should Know About Strokes.* Appleton–Century–Crofts, 1981.

As the title implies, this book is written for the families of stroke victims. In addition to a brief discussion of the various causes of strokes the book covers the various problems related to strokes, including hemiplegia, apraxia, ataxia, speech problems, visual problems, physical sensations, hearing disturbances, and general changes in bodily functions. The discussions are not lengthy but are complete enough to provide useful information. The chapters on the psychological and behavioral changes are particularly good.

INDEX

A

Abandonment, fear of, 59
Activities,
  group, 44
  individual, 44
  outside, 44
Activity chart, 44
Activity director, 35, 41, 46, 82
Activity room, 43
Adjustment to nursing home, 61, 77-86, 112
  social, 75
Administrator, 34, 40, 46, 94, 118
Admissions coordinator, 53
Adult day care center, 27-8
Aides, 35, 46
  training of, 46
Alternatives to nursing home, 12, 14, 18-29, 120-21
Alzheimer's disease, 108-09
  diagnosis of, 108
Appearance of residents, 42

B

Bathrooms, renovating, 17
Board and care homes, 19

C

Cataracts, 103
Chapel, 43
Checklist for evaluating nursing homes, 49-52, 123-29
Choosing a nursing home, 39-48
Clergy, as source of information, 9
Clothing, 73-4
Color perception, 103
Companion services, 23
Complaints, 78, 81-4, 94-5
  filing with state agency, 95
Concerns of family, 61-4
Confusion, 110-12
  techniques for dealing with, 111-12
Congregate housing, 18-19
Conservatorship, 90, 91

Continuing care arrangements, 21-2
Costs, 47-8, 87-90
Custodial trust, 92

D

Daily routine, 79-80
Decision-making process, 10-11
Dementia, 108-09
Depression, 12, 81, 107-08
  symptoms of, 107-08
Dietician, 36
Dining room, 43
Drug interactions, 11
Durable power of attorney, 93

E.C.H.O. housing, 21
Elder Cottage Housing
  Opportunity, 21
Emergency call systems, 25
Emotional needs, meeting, 85
Emotional stimulation, 85
Entry interview, 53-6
  information needed for, 53-5

F

Family, concerns of, 61-4
Family relationships, maintaining, 78
Fear of abandonment, 59
Fears, 59-61
Financial considerations, 47-8, 55, 87-90
Funeral arrangements, 55

G

Geriatric counselors, as source of information, 9
Gerontologists, 44
Glaucoma, 103
Group activities, 44
Guardianship, 90-1
Guilt, 61-4